D0603685

COMPACT *Research*

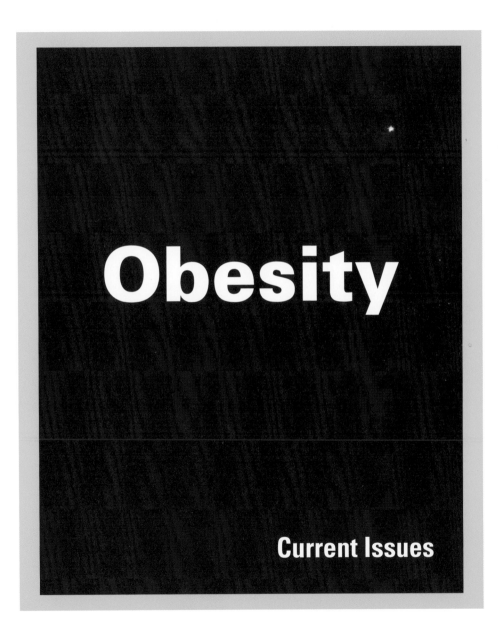

Obesity

Current Issues

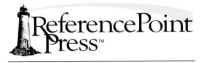

ReferencePoint
Press™

San Diego, CA

Other books in the Compact Research series include:

Drugs

Alcohol
Club Drugs
Cocaine and Crack
Hallucinogens
Heroin
Inhalants
Marijuana
Methamphetamine
Nicotine and Tobacco
Performance-Enhancing Drugs

Current Issues

Biomedical Ethics
The Death Penalty
Energy Alternatives
Free Speech
Global Warming and Climate Change
Gun Control
Illegal Immigration
National Security
Nuclear Weapons and Security
Terrorist Attacks
World Energy Crisis

Obesity

by Carrie Fredericks

Current Issues

ReferencePoint
Press™

San Diego, CA

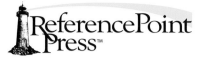

© 2008 ReferencePoint Press, Inc.

For more information, contact:
ReferencePoint Press, Inc.
PO Box 27779
San Diego, CA 92198
www.ReferencePointPress.com

Picture credits:
Maury Aaseng: 32–35, 47–50, 63–66, 79–82
AP Images: 17
Landov: 14

LIBRARY OF CONGRESS CATALOGING-IN-PUBLICATION DATA

Fredericks, Carrie.
   Obesity / by Carrie Fredericks.
      p. cm. — (Compact research series)
   Includes bibliographical references and index.
   ISBN-13: 978-1-60152-040-1 (hardback)
   ISBN-10: 1-60152-040-9 (hardback)
   1. Obesity. 2. Obesity—United States. I. Title.
   RC628.F72 2008
   616.3'98—dc22
                                                                 2007042183

Contents

Foreword

66 Where is the knowledge we have lost in information?99

—"The Rock," T.S. Eliot.

As modern civilization continues to evolve, its ability to create, store, distribute, and access information expands exponentially. The explosion of information from all media continues to increase at a phenomenal rate. By 2020 some experts predict the worldwide information base will double every 73 days. While access to diverse sources of information and perspectives is paramount to any democratic society, information alone cannot help people gain knowledge and understanding. Information must be organized and presented clearly and succinctly in order to be understood. The challenge in the digital age becomes not the creation of information, but how best to sort, organize, enhance, and present information.

ReferencePoint Press developed the *Compact Research* series with this challenge of the information age in mind. More than any other subject area today, researching current events can yield vast, diverse, and unqualified information that can be intimidating and overwhelming for even the most advanced and motivated researcher. The *Compact Research* series offers a compact, relevant, intelligent, and conveniently organized collection of information covering a variety of current and controversial topics ranging from illegal immigration to marijuana.

The series focuses on three types of information: objective single-author narratives, opinion-based primary source quotations, and facts and statistics. The clearly written objective narratives provide context and reliable background information. Primary source quotes are carefully selected and cited, exposing the reader to differing points of view. And facts and statistics sections aid the reader in evaluating perspectives. Presenting these key types of information creates a richer, more balanced learning experience.

For better understanding and convenience, the series enhances information by organizing it into narrower topics and adding design features that make it easy for a reader to identify desired content. For example, in *Compact Research: Illegal Immigration*, a chapter covering the economic impact of illegal immigration has an objective narrative explaining the various ways the economy is impacted, a balanced section of numerous primary source quotes on the topic, followed by facts and full-color illustrations to encourage evaluation of contrasting perspectives.

The ancient Roman philosopher Lucius Annaeus Seneca wrote, "It is quality rather than quantity that matters." More than just a collection of content, the *Compact Research* series is simply committed to creating, finding, organizing, and presenting the most relevant and appropriate amount of information on a current topic in a user-friendly style that invites, intrigues, and fosters understanding.

Obesity at a Glance

Prevalence

Obesity has greatly increased since the 1980s for all ages and ethnic groups.

Health Consequences

Obesity rates continue to rise despite public information campaigns that warn of health consequences such as diabetes, high blood pressure, sleep disorders, and cardiovascular disease.

Causes

Studies show that Americans exercise less and eat more even though they know that this behavior can lead to obesity.

Young People

Young people today spend many hours watching television, using computers, or playing video games, which may explain large increases in obesity among American youth.

Personal Responsibility

While many factors may contribute to obesity, personal choices concerning what to eat, how much to eat, and how much to exercise can influence the likelihood of obesity.

Treatment

Obesity treatments, which range from self-administered diets to radical life-altering surgery, have mixed results because success ultimately depends on the individual's ability and willingness to make lifestyle changes.

Prevention

Educational programs in schools and communities can teach young people about healthful eating and the importance of exercise, but families and individuals must choose to live by what they learn, which is one of the challenges of obesity prevention.

Overview

❝Obesity will be the greatest health problem of the 21st century.❞

—Christiaan Barnard, *50 Ways to a Healthy Heart*.

❝[The obesity epidemic] . . . is rooted in the changed relationships of humans to sources of sustenance and to physical activities required for survival.❞

—T. Berry Brazelton and Joshua Sparrow, quoted in Susan Okie, *Fed Up! Winning the War Against Childhood Obesity*.

Although obesity is not a new human complaint, it is only since the mid-twentieth century that the medical profession has viewed obesity as a major health issue. In America the percentage of overweight and obese individuals has dramatically increased since the 1950s, and experts have tried to explain this rise by examining the changes in culture and society that have accompanied it.

Some experts see an increase in sedentary lifestyle as one of the culprits. Post–World War II prosperity brought modern conveniences within the reach of many American families. Household appliances reduced the amount of physical exertion spent on daily chores, and the dominance of the automobile prompted more Americans to drive rather than walk. During leisure hours many families gathered around television sets instead of pursuing physical outdoor activities. As suburban life became more popular and cars became more of a necessity for Americans, the declining price of other modern conveniences made them affordable to nearly all. With the increase in the number of family cars, more people over the decades experienced a decrease in daily physical activity. For young people the birth of the video game industry in the 1970s did little to help the problem. Young people who had previously been active outside the home during the day now had reason to stay sedentary for hours at a time. Since then, the expansion of the video game market and the growth of the personal computer market and the Internet have prompted adults and young people to spend ever-increasing amounts of time in front of a video or computer screen. In 2006 the National Institute on Media and the Family reported, "Children aged 8 to 18 spend more time (44.5 hours per week) in front of computer, television, and game screens than any other activity in their lives except sleeping."[1]

> " Post–World War II prosperity brought modern conveniences within the reach of many American families. "

In addition to lack of exercise, the prevalence of diets high in carbohydrates, fats, and refined sugars have also been cited as major contributors to higher obesity rates in the last 50 years. The use of prepackaged and convenience foods, which often contain high concentrations of carbohydrates and fats, have steadily increased, starting with the first TV dinner available in 1953.

Rising Obesity Rates in the United States

According to the U.S Department of Health and Human Services the prevalence of obesity among adults aged 20 to 74 more than doubled during the period between 1960 and 2002. The National Institutes of Health (NIH) state that the obesity rate rose from 13.3 to 30.5 percent, with most of this rise happening during the past 20 years. The occurrence of morbid obesity, which is defined as being more than 100 pounds over an individual's ideal weight, increased from 0.8 percent to 4.9 percent during the same period.

The increase in obesity rates is occurring across all groups. Regardless of age, education level, gender, or socioeconomic status, obesity is steadily rising. Studies show that obesity occurs in America's minority and ethnic populations at slightly higher rates than in white Americans. Health issues brought about by obesity also occur at increased rates in minority groups. Basing its information on a 2003–2004 National Health and Nutrition Examination Survey, the Centers for Disease Control and Prevention (CDC) estimates that 66 percent of U.S. adults are overweight or obese.

This survey also found that obesity has increased among young people. Girls experienced a jump in obesity rate from 13.8 percent in 1999 to 16 percent in 2004. Boys fared even worse, their obesity rate increasing from 14 percent in 1999 to 18.2 percent in 2004. Young people are more sedentary than ever and often eat meals high in fat. Obese children and adolescents can also suffer from many of the same health issues that affect adults, including diabetes and hypertension.

What Are the Causes of Obesity?

Obesity is caused by an individual consuming more calories than the body can expend or actually needs. The main reasons for this are overeating or having a diet high in fat and calories and engaging in too little physical activity. According to weight-loss specialist Anne Collins, "Eating too many calories for our energy needs must be a major candidate for the main cause of the modern obesity epidemic."[2] If more calories are consumed, more calories need to be burned, or the excess calories are stored as fat, resulting in marked weight gain.

> "The National Institutes of Health state that the obesity rate rose from 13.3 to 30.5 percent, with most of this rise happening during the past 20 years."

Other factors are also thought to contribute to obesity. Genetics is one factor that may play a part. Because obesity often runs in families, doctors are focusing on genetic links that may explain the trend. In England, researchers have isolated a gene known as FTO that may contribute to obesity. An article in *ScienceDaily* reports, "There are two varieties of FTO, and everybody inherits two copies of the gene. But depending on which variety, you are more likely or less likely to become obese."[3]

The link between genetics and obesity has also been studied in adopted children, their birth parents, and their adoptive parents. Some of these studies suggest that genetics plays a larger role in obesity than lifestyle. According to the Memorial Weight Loss and Bariatric Surgery Center in Indiana, the weight of adoptive children has an 80 percent correlation with the weight of their genetic parents, who have had no effect on the eating habits and physical activity levels of these children.

> " Obesity is caused by an individual consuming more calories than the body can expend or actually needs. "

While genetics may contribute to obesity, some experts say genetics does not explain the growing prevalence of obesity. Stephen O'Rahilly, a biochemistry professor at Cambridge University, rejects genetics as an explanation for rising rates of obesity. "Nothing genetic explains the rise in obesity. We can't change our genes over 30 years."[4] Some of these critics suggest that the tendency of obesity to run in families may be explained by similar eating habits and lifestyle choices.

Measuring Obesity

The Body Mass Index (BMI) is a measure of body fat that is based on the height and weight of an individual. For adults, BMI is calculated by dividing a person's weight (in pounds) by the height squared (in inches) and multiplying that number by a conversion factor of 703. A BMI of 18.5 to 24.9 indicates a person of "normal weight"; an overweight BMI is 25 to 29.9; and a BMI of 30 or greater signifies obesity.

According to George A. Bray, a professor of medicine at Louisiana State University, "The body mass index (BMI) is the most practical way to evaluate the degree of overweight."[5] Because it requires only height and weight measurements, BMI is an easy tool that many physicians use to help predict future health risks and other problems associated with abnormally high amounts of body fat.

While BMI is a good indicator of body fat and obesity, some people do not fit the obesity BMI profile. Since BMI is not a direct measure of body fat, individuals with a high BMI but very low body fat are unlikely to be obese. The Centers for Disease Control and Preventon states

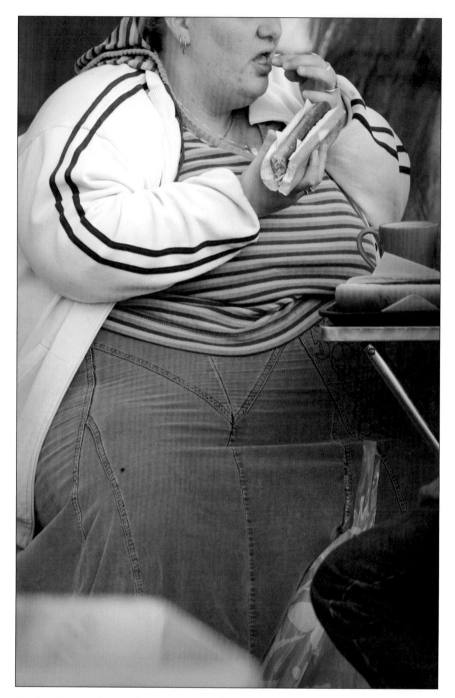

In the United States the percentage of overweight and obese individuals has dramatically increased since the 1950s. Experts have tried to explain this rise by examining the changes in culture and society that have accompanied it.

that "highly trained athletes may have a high BMI because of increased muscularity rather than increased body fatness."[6] Also, the same BMI scale is used to calculate body fat for both sexes and all ages of adults and does not take into account some differences, including the fact that women tend to have more body fat than men, and older individuals tend to have more body fat than younger people.

> **Because it requires only height and weight measurements, BMI is an easy tool that many physicians use to help predict future health risks and other problems associated with abnormally high amounts of body fat.**

While the same scale is used for all adults, the BMI scale for children and teens is based on age and sex. This is because the amount of age-appropriate body fat is different for girls and boys, and the amount of body fat a child has changes significantly as he or she grows. Percentiles are used with children and teens because of these rapid weight changes. That is, because a child's height increases through his or her growing years, what is considered a healthy weight also increases. According to the CDC, with percentiles, it is easy to show that "a 10-year-old boy with a BMI of 23 would be in the overweight category (85th percentile or greater) . . . [while] a 16-year-old boy with a BMI of 23 would be in the healthy weight category (5th percentile to less than 85th percentile)."[7]

Another measurement that is sometimes used with BMI is waist circumference. Men who measure more than 40 inches around their waists and women who measure more than 35 inches around their waists are commonly categorized as overweight. Because waist circumference is a fairly accurate indicator of abdominal fat, physicians may also use this measurement to predict the risk of obesity-related health issues such as high blood pressure and cardiovascular disease.

Obesity and Health Issues

Research shows that obesity can negatively affect an individual's health. People who are obese are at risk to develop diabetes, coronary disease, high blood pressure, arthritis, cancer, infertility, and stroke. The University of Southern California Center for Colorectal and Pelvic Floor Disorders reports that obese individuals can develop one or more serious health conditions that, if left untreated, can be fatal.

Almost daily, new links between obesity and other health conditions are uncovered. Many of these health conditions can become very serious or even fatal for the obese individual, and doctors assert that the more overweight an individual is, the greater the risks become.

Medical experts say that many of the health risks associated with obesity can be reduced by lowering one's body weight by only 5 percent. For a 250-pound individual, that is a weight reduction of only 12½ pounds. When coupled with an increase in physical activity, eating more healthy foods like fruits and vegetables and eating smaller portions can have a large impact on reducing the adverse health consequences of obesity.

Morbid Obesity

When an individual's weight significantly increases the risk of physical complications and severely impairs quality of life, he or she is considered morbidly obese. Morbid obesity occurs when a person is more than 100 pounds over ideal body weight, is 50 to 100 percent over ideal body weight, has a BMI over 40, or has a BMI over 35 with accompanying health issues resulting from being overweight. Many factors can contribute to being morbidly obese, including genetics, metabolism, and eating and physical activity habits.

> Many of these health conditions can become very serious or even fatal for the obese individual, and doctors assert that the more overweight an individual is, the greater the risks become.

Thyroid conditions can also lead to morbid obesity. The thyroid controls metabolism, which is the body's conversion of oxygen and calories into energy. When an individual's thyroid does not function properly, that person can gain large amounts of excess weight even while exercising and eating sensibly. The speed at which the body

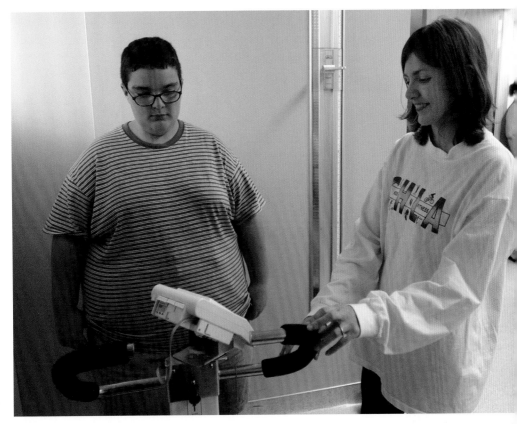

Young people today spend many hours watching television, using computers, or playing video games, which may explain large increases in obesity among American youth. This boy has developed an adult form of diabetes because of his weight.

burns up calories from the foods eaten is called the metabolic rate. The faster the metabolic rate, the more calories that are burned. With a faster metabolism an individual is less likely to be overweight or obese, and when an individual's metabolism "slows down" the body's processes slow down and weight is gained. Slowing of metabolism occurs in most people about 5 percent per decade of age.

Is Obesity a Matter of Personal Responsibility?

Many different factors and groups have been blamed for obesity. Among these are fast-food restaurants, parents who feed their children high-fat meals, and schools that have cut physical education classes to meet budgetary needs. Certain physiological conditions have also been linked to obesity, but many experts say that these conditions should not overshadow personal responsibility for obesity.

More and more, Americans live an obesity-prone lifestyle. With the prevalence of fast food, many individuals and families no longer get balanced meals that have an adequate amount of fruit, vegetables, and whole grains. The portions people eat are also larger, leading to a massive increase in calorie intake. The obesity-prone lifestyle also includes many hours of television watching, game-system playing, and computer time instead of physical activity.

> **Thyroid conditions can also lead to morbid obesity.**

Recent surveys show that despite evidence that obesity may be caused by a variety of factors, more than 50 percent of the American population believes the responsibility for obesity lies with the individual. A 2003 survey conducted for the Grocery Manufacturers of America states, "More than eight in ten Americans (83 percent) say that some personally controlled factor, either individual choice, a lack of exercise, or watching television, is responsible for obesity."[8] Where young people are concerned, survey respondents believe even more strongly that parents are largely to blame for youth obesity. In a 2006 poll conducted by the Endocrine Society and an organization called Research!America, more than 95 percent of Americans believe that responsibility for obesity lies with parents and individuals.

Obesity and the Food Pyramid

Because rates of obesity have risen so starkly since the 1980s, the U.S. government and the medical community have tried to counteract the trend. In 1992 the U.S. Department of Agriculture (USDA) created the food guide pyramid to teach Americans what portions of basic food groups an average person needs each day.

But, according to some, the pyramid has led to more obesity instead of less. The pyramid depicted carbohydrates as good and fats as bad. This has been proven not to be true, with major differences between unsaturated and saturated fats. In a *San Francisco Chronicle* article regarding food pyramids, Michael Jacobson, executive director of the Center for

Science in the Public Interest, states that in the food pyramid, "there's no distinction between a cheeseburger and lentil soup."[9]

To counteract some of the criticism of the pyramid and to try to help curb the rising obesity trend in the United States, the USDA unveiled a new pyramid in 2005. The aims of the new MyPyramid, which offers more of a personalized eating plan, are to help individuals "make smart choices from every food group; find your balance between food and physical activity; get the most nutrition out of your calories; stay within your daily calorie needs."[10] In addition to developing a new pyramid for adults, the USDA has also developed a MyPyramid for kids, aimed at 6- to 11-year-olds, with the hope of helping youths make better food choices and be more active.

How Should Obesity Be Treated?

Many treatment options are available to the more than 60 percent of the U.S. population that is overweight or obese. One of the most common options is to limit the amount of food being consumed, or to diet. When a body takes in fewer calories while expending the same energy as before, the body will lose weight. Another option is to increase the amount of physical activity. According to one expert, "By burning a hundred more calories each day, a person can lose up to ten pounds each year."[11] Combining increased activity with decreased calorie intake can have a large positive impact on an individual's weight. While these two options sound very straightforward, the reality is that many people cannot control their weight through diet and exercise alone.

> " Recent surveys show that despite evidence that obesity may be caused by a variety of factors, more than 50 percent of the American population believes the responsibility for obesity lies with the individual. "

Drug treatments are another option to counteracting obesity. One of the medications used for obesity reduces the feeling of hunger, and another prevents fat (from the foods we eat) from being processed and absorbed by the small intestine. This allows the fats to be eliminated from the body without the calories being absorbed.

Surgery is another, more drastic option. Bariatric surgery, as it is known, includes several surgical procedures that can be used to control an individual's weight. These procedures range from simply making the stomach physically smaller to more radical procedures that involve a major portion of the digestive system. In most cases, bariatric surgery is performed only on people who are morbidly obese, or more than 100 pounds overweight.

Future Outlook

Obesity rates have been rising steadily in the last 50 years and show no signs of slowing down any time soon. Some states, such as Kentucky, predict a significant rise in obesity in the next several years. As one researcher notes, "Kentucky's obesity rate will likely exceed 36 percent . . . by 2015."[12] Many other states predict similar increases in obesity in coming years.

Research into obesity, already a growing area of study, will continue. The National Institutes of Health Web site, Clinicaltrials.gov, lists at least 95 ongoing studies related to children and obesity, and the NIH has also initiated a study to look at the benefits and risks of bariatric surgery for adolescents.

One of the problems with treating obesity is that the statistical data to back up certain treatment options are not always available. The CDC and the NIH, along with obesity research centers at universities across the nation, hope to gather much more information in the coming years to help alleviate the growing obesity epidemic.

What Are the Causes of Obesity?

> **Weight gain and obesity are caused by consuming more calories than the body needs—most commonly by eating a diet high in fat and calories, being sedentary or both.**
>
> —Obesity in America, "Causes of Obesity."

> **The increase in obesity over the past 30 years has been fueled by a complex interplay of environmental, social, economic, and behavioral factors, acting on a background of genetic susceptibility.**
>
> —National Institutes of Health, "About NIH Obesity Research."

Obesity is a complex problem, in that it has many causes. Some are tied to individual behavior and personal choice. Poor eating habits and lack of exercise, for example, can lead to obesity. Other causes stem from physiological conditions that may have existed from birth. A person's genetic makeup, for instance, might make one person more likely than another to develop obesity. According to the National Center for Biotechnology Information, "Evidence suggests that obesity has more than one cause: genetic, environmental, psychological and other factors may all play a part."[13] These various causes are the subject of much interest and study because the key to eliminating obesity is understanding what causes it in the first place.

Eating Choices

Poor eating habits can contribute to obesity. The U.S. Department of Agriculture states that a healthy diet should include grains, especially whole grains; vegetables, especially dark green varieties; fruit in any form (canned, fresh, frozen, or dried); milk and milk-based foods like cheese and yogurt; lean meats, poultry, and beans; and oils and fats, which should be eaten sparingly. A healthy diet should contain an average of 2,000 calories per day, including 65g total fats, 300mg cholesterol, and 2,400mg sodium.

In contrast to this is the average American diet, which has an excess of fats, sugars, and calories. Prepackaged foods and fast foods, which are a large part of the American diet, are generally laden with fat and cholesterol. For example, a meal from McDonald's containing a Big Mac sandwich, a large order of french fries, and a 32-ounce cola contains over 1,400 calories, almost 75 percent of the recommended daily calorie intake for adults. The sandwich alone contains 540 calories, including 29g of fat and 1,040mg of sodium, meaning that one sandwich gives almost 50 percent of the recommended fat and sodium totals.

> These various causes are the subject of much interest and study because the key to eliminating obesity is understanding what causes it in the first place.

The Centers for Disease Control and Prevention reports that prepackaged and processed foods are more accessible and convenient than ever before. Some of these are even sold as healthy alternatives even though they may not be healthier or a good alternative to other foods. The CDC states, "Choosing many foods from these areas may contribute to an excessive calorie intake. Some foods are marketed as healthy, low fat, or fat-free, but may contain more calories than the fat containing food they are designed to replace. It is important to read food labels for nutritional information and eat in moderation."[14]

Lack of Exercise

Physical activity has become nonexistent in the lives of many Americans. The CDC reports that 25 percent of the American population is sedentary, meaning they get little or no exercise. Using Census Bureau figures, this translates into more than 74,849,000 Americans who reported no physical activities in their leisure time.

Even walking has become obsolete. Most Americans today rely heavily on cars to get where they need to go, no matter how near or far the destination. According to the Rhode Island Department of Health, "Communities are built in ways that require people to use cars to get around."[15] Corner grocers and nearby clothing shops are a thing of the past. Downtown shopping areas that people walked to have been replaced by malls that they have to drive to. Walking just about anywhere has decreased dramatically in the last two decades. Many young people no longer walk to and from school, even if that school is only blocks from their homes.

> **Physical activity has become nonexistent in the lives of many Americans.**

Young people also spend much less time outdoors playing sports and riding bikes than they once did. Many now spend hours at a time watching television, playing video games, or using the computer. The average American household has the television on for at least seven hours per day. A survey done by NPD Group, a market research firm, shows that young people aged 6–17 (especially boys) are spending a significant amount of time playing video and computer games. According to the survey, one-half of the survey respondents play 5 hours per week or less, but the other half are much heavier users, averaging up to 16 hours or more per week. This translates to an average of up to 2 hours per day playing video or computer games.

Overeating

Overeating is widely viewed as another cause of obesity. While the U.S. government recommends a diet with an average of 2,000 calories per day, the average American eats about 2,700 calories per day. This is about 500 to 700 more calories per day than the average American ate in the 1950s.

Blue Cross Blue Shield of Massachusetts states that an increase of just 150 calories per day can add 15 pounds per year to an individual's weight.

One of the main reasons for overeating is portion size. In restaurants, portion sizes have increased dramatically, especially in fast-food establishments. "Super-sizing" fast-food meals is commonplace—what used to be called a large drink is now a small, and what used to be called adult-sized is now child-sized. This leads to increased calorie consumption, which requires increased physical activity to balance out the extra food intake or the individual gains weight.

> One of the main reasons for overeating is portion size.

Another cause of overeating may by physiological. Researchers say the hormonelike substance called dopamine (a neurotransmitter) is involved in behavior motivation and reward. When individuals encounter foods that they are accustomed to eating, especially in the case of those with high fat or sugar content, an increase in dopamine levels occurs in the brain, which interprets this as pleasure or a reward. In obese individuals, the brain may have fewer receptors to monitor the dopamine levels. This means that an obese person needs to eat more food to reach a feeling of satisfaction. In studying dopamine levels, recent research has shown that "in obesity, some people may be at greater risk for compulsive eating because they may be overly sensitive to the rewards to food."[16] These individuals may be more susceptible to food cravings and overeating.

Genetics

The connection between obesity and genetics has received a lot of attention in recent years. Some researchers believe that as much as 70 percent of obesity risk is tied to genetics. According to Barry Levin, a neurologist at New Jersey Medical School, "Your set point [an individual's constant weight] is genotype-specific, meaning its tied to your genetic template, and it's very difficult to change."[17]

One of the connections between genetics and obesity is the storage of body fat. Every human stores fat, usually in the middle area because it is easier for the body to carry it there. Researchers think that excess body fat is genetically programmed in some obese individuals. This means they may begin life with a body type that retains more fat, is more sensitive to high-fat and high-sugar foods, and is less able to get rid of excess weight.

Genes also influence appetite and how much food it takes to feel full. This is mainly done through the hypothalamus, the area of the brain linking the nervous system with the endocrine system. This region of the brain responds to sensory inputs like taste and smell and tells the body whether it is hungry or full. It also regulates the burning of fat through metabolism. If variations exist in the genes that control the hypothalamus or any of the accompanying processes, an individual could have a problem controlling how much food he or she eats and how much fat is burned.

Gender

Studies show that women are more likely to become obese than men. The American Obesity Association reports that 62 percent of women aged 20 to 74 are overweight, and at least 50 percent of those overweight women are obese. For men, 67 percent are overweight, but less than half that number are obese.

One explanation for a higher rate of obesity in women is that generally women have more fat tissue and men have more muscle tissue. Muscle tissue uses more energy than fat tissue. St. Vincent Health, a member of the Ascension Health System, states, "Men have more muscle than women, and burn 10 percent to 20 percent more calories than women do at rest. For this reason, women are more likely to be obese."[18]

Higher rates of obesity have also been tied to childbirth. During pregnancy, most women gain an average of 30 pounds and tend to keep some of that weight after birth. Postpregnancy, the average woman weighs roughly 5 pounds more than she did before pregnancy and commonly maintains that extra weight. In many cases, this extra weight gain is compounded by more than one pregnancy.

> **Higher rates of obesity have also been tied to childbirth.**

Menopause has also been shown to have an effect on the development of obesity. After menopause a woman's ovaries stop producing the hormone estrogen. This hormone is critical in female development. In a study conducted at the University of Texas Health Science Center at San Antonio, results suggested that the loss of estrogen after menopause may play a significant role in causing obesity.

Psychological and behavioral problems are often tied to obesity. Many people eat in response to emotional distress, including depression, boredom, or anger. The Cleveland Clinic's Bariatric Surgery Department reports, "While most overweight people have no more psychological disturbances than people at their normal weight, about 30 percent of the people who seek treatments for serious weight problems have difficulties with binge eating."[19] Binge eating is defined as consuming large quantities of food in a short amount of time. These episodes can be uncontrolled and followed by feelings of guilt, anger, and depression. This in turn can lead to more binge eating and can be an unending cycle for many obese individuals.

> " This means that in many cases an obese individual will not have the body's natural appetite-suppressing mechanism to help control weight gain. "

Medications for psychological disorders can also contribute to obesity. In some cases, drugs prescribed for psychiatric conditions can slow how quickly the body burns calories. Other psychiatric medications have side effects that may include appetite stimulation, which causes an individual to eat more food more often than they normally would. Other side effects include water retention, in which the body's tissues hold on to more water, causing weight gain.

For the obese individual, food and emotions are often inextricably tied together. These emotions can be both negative and positive, but both situations can adversely affect an individual's weight and health.

Leptin

Recent research has shown that for some individuals, the hormone leptin may have a large influence on obesity. Leptin is formed and released from an individual's fat cells and functions to suppress the appetite and increase energy output. Receptors in the brain detect the amount of leptin in the body.

The problem begins when mutations occur in leptin. Changes can happen that cause the whole system to go haywire. This can cause people to constantly feel hungry, which leads to excessive weight gain.

Many studies are being conducted on mice to help understand the possible connection between leptin and obesity. In an Oregon study obese individuals have been shown to have a lesser reponse to the leptin hormone. The amount of leptin rises as an individual gains weight, and these rising leptin levels should help decrease the amount of food that that individual wishes to eat. *ScienceDaily*, a health information provider, remarks, "However, high levels of leptin, which can be found in severely overweight individuals, can lead to leptin resistance. Leptin resistance means that the body no longer responds to the hormone's weight suppressing effects."[20] This means that in many cases an obese individual will not have the body's natural appetite-suppressing mechanism to help control weight gain.

Leptin has other effects on the body besides appetite and energy control. Research is now being done on how leptin may be linked to obesity-related cardiovascular disease, asthma, and breast cancer.

Other Causes

In some instances, other illnesses can cause obesity. Cushing's syndrome is one example. This syndrome occurs when the body produces large levels of the hormone cortisol. The Endocrine and Metabolic Diseases Information Service, part of the National Institutes of Health, reports, "Symptoms vary, but most people have upper body obesity, rounded face, increased fat around the neck, and thinning arms and legs. Children tend to be obese with slowed growth rates."[21]

Drugs such as steroids can also contribute to obesity. Steroids are often used by individuals with autoimmune disorders like Crohn's Disease or multiple sclerosis (MS) to control inflammation. These steroids often cause a person to put on a large amount of weight in a very short time. When an individual is gradually taken off the steroids his or her weight often decreases. But many people never lose the entire amount of weight that was gained from the use of these medications.

The causes of obesity are myriad and complex. Many different factors lead to obesity. In some cases it may be one overwhelming factor, while in other cases several circumstances can lead to the same obesity result.

What Are the Causes of Obesity?

66 In most cases, the genes involved in weight gain do not directly cause obesity but rather they increase the susceptibility to fat gain in subjects exposed to an environment characterized by an abundance of food and limited physical activity. 99

> Thomas P. LaFontaine and Jeffrey L. Roitman, "Lifestyle Management of Obesity: Etiology of Obesity," 2007. wwwvhct.org/case2500/etiology.htm.

LaFontaine is Manager of Boone Hospital Center in Columbia, Missouri and Roitman is Director of Cardiac Rehabilitation at Baptist Medical Center and Research Medical Center in Kansas City, Missouri.

66 We know from twin studies that approximately 50 percent of the risk for both addiction and obesity is genetic. 99

> —Nora D. Volkow, quoted in Kristin Leutwyler Ozelli, "This Is Your Brain on Food," *Scientific American*, vol. 297, no. 3, September 2007.

Volkow is the director of the National Institute on Drug Abuse.

Bracketed quotes indicate conflicting positions.

* Editor's Note: While the definition of a primary source can be narrowly or broadly defined, for the purposes of Compact Research, a primary source consists of: 1) results of original research presented by an organization or researcher; 2) eyewitness accounts of events, personal experience, or work experience; 3) first-person editorials offering pundits' opinions; 4) government officials presenting political plans and/or policies; 5) representatives of organizations presenting testimony or policy.

“We lead busy lives, eat fast, and choose television or computer over exercise.”

—Morefocus, "Causes of Obesity and Weight Gain," 2007. www.obesityfocused.com.

Morefocus provides information on a variety of health-care-related topics.

“You're built as a machine to ingest food and ingest palatable foods. It's going to take some work to stop that when the food is freely available.”

—Allen Levine, quoted in Rob Schmitz, "Obesity and the Brain," Minnesota Public Radio, June 2, 2003 and April 11, 2005. http://news.minnesota.publicradio.org.

Levine researches the effects of sugar and other substances on rats' brains at the Veterans' Affairs Hospital in Minneapolis.

“Biology and genes are the biggest contributing factor, with obesity being the most likely trait to be inherited after height.”

—Tony Stephenson, "Obesity Lecture Sees Heavyweight Researchers Battle It Out," Imperial College of London, May 25, 2006. www.imperial.ac.uk.

Stephenson is the press officer for the Imperial College of Science, Technology, and Medicine, which was part of the University of London until July 2007, when it became an independent university. The Imperial College is a scientific, engineering, and medical research and teaching facility.

“Obesity experts consider the Western lifestyle to be the single largest contributing factor to obesity.”

—M. Sara Rosenthal, *The Type 2 Diabetes Sourcebook for Women.* New York: McGraw-Hill, 2005.

Rosenthal is the author of more than 25 health books and is assistant professor of bioethics at the University of Kentucky College of Medicine.

❝ Our bodies' tendencies to become obese and to develop type 2 diabetes are affected not only by our genes and our lifestyle, but also by our early development. **❞**

—Francine R. Kaufman, *Diabesity*. New York: Bantam 2005.

Kaufman is the author of more than 150 medical articles and the head of the Center for Diabetes, Endocrinology and Metabolism at Children's Hospital in Los Angeles, California.

❝ It's well accepted that reduced physical activity and fast food are linked to obesity. But the evidence that these are the *main* causes of obesity is 'largely circumstantial.' **❞**

—David B. Allison, quoted in CBSNews.com, "Study Suggests 10 New Obesity Causes," June 27, 2006. www.cbsnews.com.

Allison is director of the University of Alabama at Birmingham's clinical nutrition research center.

❝ The stress of life at low educational and socioeconomic levels is a direct cause of obesity. **❞**

—Elissa Epel, quoted in Mary Ferguson, "A Growing Problem: Race, Class and Obesity Among American Women," 2007. http://jounalism.nyu.edu.

Epel studies the relationship between stress and fat distribution and growth hormones at the University of California at San Francisco.

❝ There are typically three times as many supermarkets per capita in upper- and middle-income neighborhoods as there are in low-income neighborhoods. **❞**

—Morgan Spurlock, *Don't Eat This Book: Fast Food and the Supersizing of America*. New York: G.P. Putnam's Sons, 2005.

Spurlock is a writer and documentary filmmaker. He is known for his film *Super Size Me*.

Facts and Illustrations

What Are the Causes of Obesity?

- According to the American Obesity Association, approximately 127 million adults in the United States are overweight, **60 million obese**, and 9 million severely obese.

- People who get **20 to 30 minutes of exercise** most days are less likely to be obese.

- By the year 2000 more than **26 percent of adults** reported no leisure-time physical activity.

- Overall, more than **430 genes**, markers, and chromosomal regions have been associated or linked with human obesity phenotypes.

- Obesity affects **10 to 25 percent** of the European population and nearly 33 percent of the U.S. population.

- Most dietary research suggests that people should limit the amount of fatty foods they consume to less than **30 percent** of their daily energy consumption.

- An estimated **300,000 deaths** can be attributed to obesity.

- Overweight adolescents have a **70 percent chance** of becoming overweight or obese adults. This increases to 80 percent if one or more parent is overweight or obese.

Obesity Across America

According to a report from the Trust for America's Health, obesity rates have increased in over 30 states and remained steady in all other states. The highest rate of obesity was over 30 percent for Mississippi. Colorado has the lowest rate at 17.6 percent.

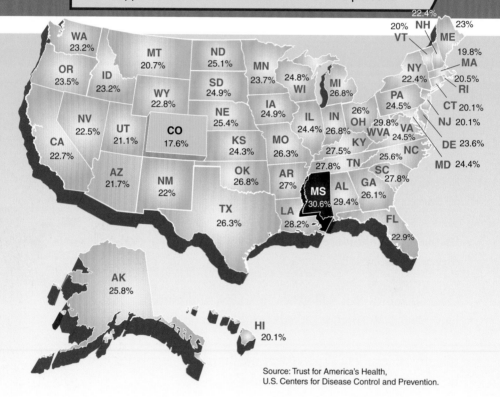

Source: Trust for America's Health,
U.S. Centers for Disease Control and Prevention.

- Obese individuals have a **10 to 50 percent increase** in the risk of death from any cause, compared with normal-weight individuals.

- Teens average an **extra 300 calories** over the recommended daily amount.

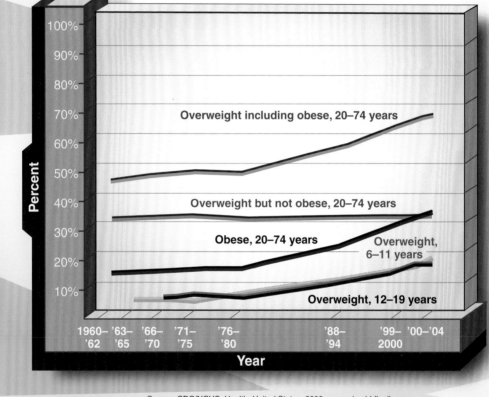

Overweight and Obesity by Age in the United States, 1960–2004

Obesity and overweight have been on the rise for all age groups in the last 25 years. Overweight is defined as having a body mass index (BMI) of 25–29.9, while anyone with a BMI of 30 or more is considered obese.

Source: CDC/NCHS, Health, United States, 2006. www.win.niddk.nih.gov.

- The fast-food industry serves almost **33 percent** of American adults every day.

- An excess of **100 calories per day** (about 60 percent of a 12 oz. can of soda) will add up to 10 extra pounds in one year.

Obesity in Americans over Age 50

For adults over age 50 the rate of obesity is greater for the 51–69 age group than it is for the above 70 age group. The individuals with lower income and less education also have a higher rate of obesity. The percentage of obesity in adults over age 50 is more than 20 percent regardless of other determining factors such as race or ethnicity, income levels, and amount of education. The percentage of obese individuals declines in people above age 70, but then it only declines to 17 percent.

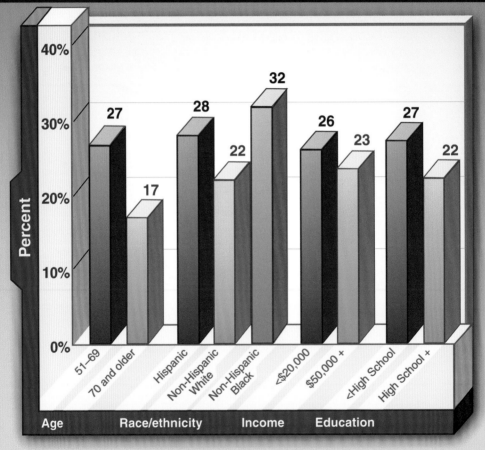

Source: Center on an Aging Society, Georgetown University, "Obesity Among Older Americans," July 2003.

Contributors to Obesity

Although many people believe that obesity is due mainly to an individual's personal choices, many different factors like genetics, gender, and socioeconomic status can contribute to obesity.

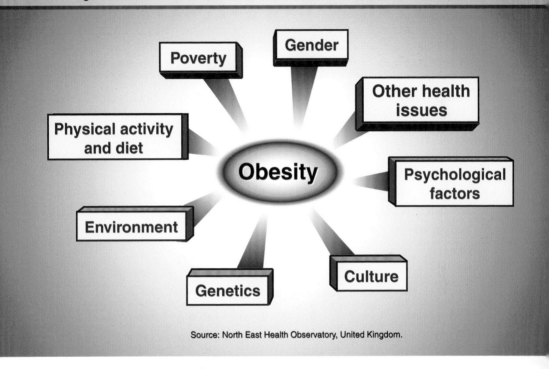

Source: North East Health Observatory, United Kingdom.

- Eating breakfast reduces the risk of obesity by more than **35 percent**.

- If both parents in a family are obese, **66 percent** of their children will be obese.

- In 1981 **Better Homes and Gardens'** basic chocolate chip cookie recipe yielded 72 cookies. In 2007 the same basic recipe yields 60 cookies.

How Can Obesity Be Prevented?

66 The most important thing a person can do to combat obesity is to prevent obesity before it develops. 99

— Obesity in America, "Obesity Treatment with Medications."

66 In theory, all it should take to prevent the problem is for people to eat less and move more—in other words to become personally responsible for maintaining a healthy lifestyle. 99

— Francine R. Kaufman, *Diabesity*.

Because so many cases of obesity are rooted in lifestyle choices and dietary habits, prevention is possible. But just because it is possible does not mean it is easy. Changing one's lifestyle—or getting others to change their lifestyle—requires determination and commitment from many different sources. Diet, activity, and lifestyle can all play a role in preventing obesity, but not by themselves. If an individual goes on a diet but does not change his or her sedentary lifestyle, obesity may still occur. And young people who try to eat well but get no physical activity may still be at risk of developing obesity. Parents, individuals, consumer groups, industries, manufacturers, communities, and the government can all help in the prevention of obesity.

Maintaining a Healthy Weight

Making sure the number of calories burned equals the number of calories consumed keeps an individual at a certain weight. A balanced and healthy diet along with daily physical activity is key to maintaining a healthy weight. According to the U.S. Department of Agriculture, there are five main food groups: grains, vegetables, fruits, milk, and meat/beans. The USDA advises, "For good health, eat a variety of foods from each group every day."[22] The milk group includes yogurt and cheese; the meat and beans group includes poultry, fish, eggs, dry beans, and nuts.

> A balanced and healthy diet along with daily physical activity is key to maintaining a healthy weight.

Portion sizes are also instrumental in a healthy diet. In the last 20 years, portion sizes have increased dramatically. So even if an individual is eating the right kinds of foods, eating too much of these foods still leads to an increase in the amount of calories consumed. The Centers for Disease Control and Prevention reports, "Choosing a variety of healthy foods in the correct portion sizes is helpful for achieving and maintaining a healthy weight."[23]

Water also plays an important role in weight maintenance. The Harvard School of Public Health recommends that women consume 90 to 120 ounces of water daily. For men, the recommended totals are 120 ounces of beverages daily with 25 ounces of water from foods. Low water intake can affect kidney function. If the kidneys are not functioning properly then the liver picks up what the kidneys cannot process. Since one of the main functions of the liver is to metabolize fat into energy, the low water intake can lead to weight gain or the decreased ability to maintain a healthy weight.

The Sleep Cycle

Getting proper amounts of sleep can also help prevent obesity. Many Americans, both adults and young people, do not get enough sleep. The average person needs 7 to 9 hours of sleep per night but gets less than 7 hours per night, according to the National Sleep Foundation.

Lack of sleep can lead a person to feel tired during the day, making them less inclined to be physically active. This lack of physical activity can lead to weight gain. As an individual gains extra weight, it can become more difficult to get a good night's sleep, which leads back to less activity during the day. This cycle can be hard to break.

Getting an adequate amount of sleep can help prevent obesity in another way. According to the National Sleep Foundation, "Insufficient sleep affects growth hormone secretion that is linked to obesity; as the amount of the hormone secretion decreases, the chance for weight gain increases."[24]

Sleep deprivation can also raise the levels of the hormone grehlin, which is very important in appetite regulation. Elevated levels of this hormone prompt an individual to increase food intake, which would normally result in lower grehlin levels. In obese individuals, food intake does not always cause the grehlin levels to decrease, and so these individuals continue to want more food. Getting enough sleep each night can be an important ingredient in the overall prevention of obesity.

Children and Obesity Prevention

For children, parents and family are one of the main components of obesity prevention. Most children mimic what their parents do. If a parent has an unhealthy diet and gets little exercise, then the chances are much greater that children in that household will also eat poorly and not exercise. It is almost impossible for a child to eat healthily if the parent does not, so the only way to correct this is to have the whole household eating healthy, well-balanced meals.

> It is almost impossible for a child to eat healthily if the parent does not, so the only way to correct this is to have the whole household eating healthy, well-balanced meals.

A University of Missouri at Columbia study done between 1998 and 2002 with nearly 8,500 school-age children has shown that eating meals at the dinner table instead of in front of the TV can help prevent obesity. In a Reuters Health article, author Anne Harding reports, "The fewer meals children ate each week with their families, the more likely they were to put on excess pounds."[25] In the same article, study author Sara Gable is quoted as writing, "Children rely on parents to initiate such things as family mealtimes and to set limits on children's TV time. . . . Teaching children about healthy habits requires the whole family's involvement; children are not going to learn these things on their own."[26]

Another way to prevent childhood obesity is to keep children active in the summer. A recent study has shown that young people can gain as much or more weight in the summer than they do during the school year. Researchers are not sure why this happens, but they believe that for some students, the amount of physical activity drops off dramatically at the end of the school year. Many young people, if not given opportunities to be physically active, will choose not to be. Citing this study, Reuters Health reports that researchers "speculate that a lack of structure has something to do with it. When children are in school, the researchers note, they have limited chances to snack and typically have designated times for exercise. . . . In the summer, however, many children may eat when they want or spend time in front of the TV instead of moving."[27]

> **Raising public awareness about obesity problems and risks not only allows people to make better choices for preventing obesity, it also allows them to have a better understanding of their overall health.**

Teaching People About Healthy Lifestyles

Educating people about proper nutrition and exercise can go a long way in preventing obesity. Once people have the tools they need they can make good choices. Raising public awareness about obesity problems and risks not only allows people to make better choices for preventing obesity, it also allows them to have a better understanding of their overall health.

One example of a multifaceted obesity education program is the CDC's Nutrition and Physical Activity Program to Prevent Obesity and Other Chronic Diseases. Administered in conjunction with 28 of the 50 states, the program works "to build lasting and comprehensive efforts to address obesity and other chronic diseases through a variety of nutrition and physical activity strategies."[28] Some of these strategies include "Fruits and Veggies—More Matters," an initiative designed to help increase daily consumption of fruits and vegetables; the Youth Media Campaign VERB, designed to increase physical activity in youth and help parents and educators understand the importance of physical activity; and ACES (Active Community Environments Initiative), designed to promote walking, bicycling, and accessible recreation facilities.

Many states also offer their own nutrition and physical activity programs. Massachusetts, for example, offers the 5-2-1 Go! Program. This program stresses 5 servings of fruits and vegetables daily; limiting total television, computer, and video game time to 2 hours daily; and getting at least one hour of physical activity every day. Every education program is one more step forward in the prevention of obesity.

Education in the Workplace

Workplaces are often a good starting point for obesity prevention. The American College of Occupational and Environmental Medicine has a list of recommendations regarding obesity prevention in the workplace. Both major projects like wellness centers and simpler ideas like offering educational materials on healthier food choices can be part of obesity prevention.

Some individuals believe that workplaces should be much more responsible for the overall health of their workers, especially regarding obesity. This is in the best interests of employers as well as employees. Studies have shown a relationship between increased obesity rates and increased short-term disability rates. In her article "Reducing Obesity in the Workplace" Charlene Rennick states that corporate wellness plans should focus on obesity because "it is the most common, most expensive and least addressed disease among the workforce today."[29] She also states that to help address the obesity issue, wellness plans should include options for healthier workplace choices like better vending machine foods and better cafeteria selections.

> Over 39 million workdays are lost every year due to obesity.

Another reason for workplace prevention of obesity is the relationship between physical and mental health. When employees do not feel well physically, they also might not perform their jobs to the best of their abilities. The U.S. Social Security Administration states that obesity increases the risk of developing physical impairments that would affect an individual's ability to complete everyday work tasks. Over 39 million workdays are lost every year due to obesity.

Holistic nutritionist Mike Adams seems to sum up the workplace prevention idea when he states, "The employer can make a huge difference here by encouraging employees to get out and take a walk, take a break, or get some natural sunlight on their skin. They can also provide options in terms of healthy nutrition."[30]

How Can Obesity Be Prevented?

66 **Who should pay to promote healthy living? There must be multiple payers, including individuals, the insurance industry, employers, unions, and the private sector via philanthropy. But the predominant payer must remain the government.** 99

—Francine R. Kaufman, *Diabesity*. New York: Bantam, 2005.

Kaufman is head of the Center for Diabetes, Endocrinology and Metabolism at Children's Hospital in Los Angeles, California, and professor of pediatrics at the University of Southern California Keck School of Medicine.

....

66 **Prevention is clearly more cost effective than treatment, both in terms of economic and personal costs.** 99

—International Union of Nutritional Sciences, "The Global Challenge of Obesity and the International Obesity Task Force," October 2002. www.iuns.org.

The International Union of Nutritional Scientists promotes research and development and information dissemination in the field of nutritional science.

....

* Editor's Note: While the definition of a primary source can be narrowly or broadly defined, for the purposes of Compact Research, a primary source consists of: 1) results of original research presented by an organization or researcher; 2) eyewitness accounts of events, personal experience, or work experience; 3) first-person editorials offering pundits' opinions; 4) government officials presenting political plans and/or policies; 5) representatives of organizations presenting testimony or policy.

❝Serving small portions to young children is often the best way for them to learn to eat only until satisfied, instead of overeating.❞

—Meals Matter, "Making Sense of Portion Sizes," August 14, 2007. www.mealsmatter.org.

Meals Matter, sponsored by the Dairy Council of California, offers interactive tools to help make healthy meals and healthy food choices.

❝Studies have shown that rigidly restricting children's access to certain foods focuses more attention on these foods and increases children's desire to eat them.❞

—Williams Sears et al., *The Healthiest Kid in the Neighborhood.* Boston: Little, Brown, 2006.

The Sears family has authored many books on the subjects of child rearing and children's health.

❝Reducing the prevalence of this disease will take a cross-cultural collective effort of health promotion planning between all levels of North American consumerism and corporate marketing to make obesity an unnecessary part of the American lifestyle.❞

—Charlene Rennick, "Reducing Obesity in the Workplace," May 15, 2007. www.americanchronicle.com.

Rennick is an author and the editor of three corporate health promotion and wellness Web sites.

66 Americans spend ⅓ of their lives or more at their work-place. As a result, the workplace is a major influencing factor on the health of all Americans, and it is the work-place where we need to start making some long-term changes that support optimum health and prevent chronic disease.99

—Mike Adams, "Employers Must Take On Some Responsibility for Employees' Health in Order to Prevent Obesity and Chronic Disease," *NewsTarget*, August 5, 2004. www.newstarget.com.

Adams is a health author, nutritionist, and executive director of the Consumer Wellness Center.

66 Corporations and organizations have a vested interest in their employees' lifestyles, since what they do off the job also affects how they perform on the job.99

—B.J. Gallagher, quoted in Lori Widmer, "Fat Chance: Obesity in the Workplace," June 2005.

Gallagher is coauthor of *Who Are "They" Anyway*, a book about personal account-ability.

66 Obesity is likely to continue to increase, and if noth-ing is done, it will soon become the leading prevent-able cause of death in the United States.99

—May Beydoun, quoted in Reuters Health, "Three in Four in US Will Be Overweight by 2015," July 19, 2007. www.shapingamericashealth.com.

Beydoun was part of a team of researchers at Johns Hopkins University in Balti-more, Maryland, that studied Americans' future weight and behavior.

66 An environment that promotes healthy weight is one that encourages consumption of nutritious foods in reasonable portions and regular physical activity. A healthy environment is important for all individuals to prevent and treat obesity and maintain weight loss. **99**

—American Obesity Association, "Causes of Obesity," May 2, 2005. www.obesityusa.org.

The American Obesity Association is an obesity education and advocacy organization.

66 Our current environment does not encourage healthy lifestyles, and it will take time to create one that does. **99**

—James O. Hill, "Addressing the Environment to Reduce Obesity," National Institutes of Health, 2007.

Hill is director of the Center for Human Nutrition at the University of Colorado Health Sciences Center.

66 Only when Americans feel the countervailing cost of being fat in their daily lives will they begin to step out of the obesity epidemic. **99**

—Greg Critser, *Fat Land: How Americans Became the Fattest People in the World*. Boston: Houghton Mifflin, 2003.

Critser is a California-based journalist covering medical, health, and nutrition topics.

Facts and Illustrations

How Can Obesity Be Prevented?

- According to the American Academy of Pediatrics, **only 15 percent** of teenagers sleep the suggested amount of 8.5 hours on school nights.

- The Trust for America's Health reports that obesity rates **continue to rise in 31 states**.

- According to the National Institute on Media and the Family, children who watch more than three hours of television per day are **50 percent more likely to be obese** than children who watch less than two hours.

- The New York State Department of Health reports that the number of obese children **has tripled in the past 30 years**.

- The U.S. Department of Agriculture recommends an average of **1,800–2,400 calories per day for females** and 2,200–3,000 calories per day for males, depending on an individual's level of activity.

- A serving of fruit or vegetables is about the **size of a fist**.

- For women, when BMI exceeds 30 the risk of death related to obesity **increases 50 percent**. More than **33 percent** of women in the United States are obese, according to the American Obesity Association.

Americans Eating Out More Often

Food choices have much to do with an individual's weight. Convenience, health, cost, time elements, and taste all factor into which foods someone chooses. According to the USDA, in the past 40 years Americans have greatly increased the amount of money spent eating out. In 1962 less than 28 percent of total food expenditures were used to eat out. More than 40 years later that percentage has increased to more than 50 percent.

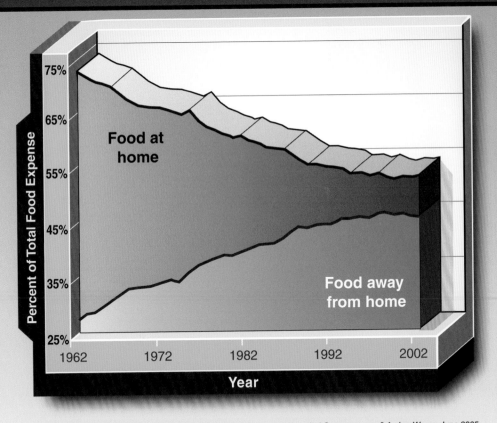

Source: USDA, Fred Kuchler et al., "Obesity Policy and the Law of Unintended Consequences," *Amber Waves*, June 2005.

- The average American has had an average weight gain of **1 to 2 pounds per year** in the last 7 to 10 years, according to Dr. James Hill.

Childhood Obesity Percentages

Obesity is becoming more of a problem in children, especially in minorities. Fifteen percent of all children and 25 percent of Hispanic and African American children are overweight. The National Institute of Environmental Health Sciences reports that as these obese children become obese adults, complications and health risks of this disease have the potential to rise dramatically.

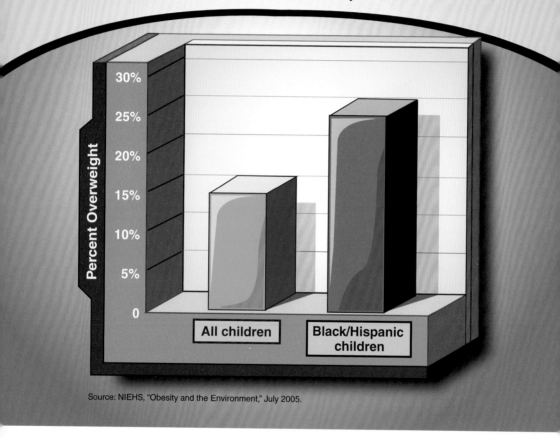

Source: NIEHS, "Obesity and the Environment," July 2005.

- The National Institutes of Health report that 20 years ago the average cup of coffee was made with whole milk and sugar, was 8 ounces, and had 45 calories. Today the average cup of take-out coffee is made with steamed whole milk and flavored syrup, **is 16 ounces, and has 350 calories**.

Liquids Compose over 20 Percent of America's Diet

A study commissioned by the Milk Processor Education Program has shown that for most people, more than 20 percent of total calories come from liquids. This means that people trying to lose weight or control weight must pay attention to what they are drinking in addition to what they are eating. The bottom pie chart gives a breakdown of liquid consumption in 2004. Carbonated soft drinks is the highest at 32 percent.

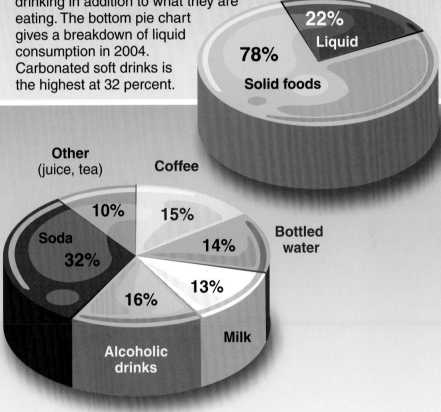

Source: Mark Weintraub, "Liquids Make Up 22 Percent of American Diet," *Consumer Health News*, January 8, 2007.

- Between the ages of 10 and 18, activity levels fall **more than 60 percent for girls**.

Portion Comparisons

Portion sizes have increased greatly in the past five decades. It is often hard to know what is the correct amount of food. Visualizing proper portion sizes using everyday objects can help keep an individual on track for eating the recommended amount of a certain type of food. The table below shows objects that can be used to aid in portion control. Each measurement equals one serving.

	3 oz. meat
	1 oz. cheese
	Medium potato
	2 Tbs. peanut butter
	1/2 cup pasta
	Average size bagel

Source: American Cancer Society.

Is Obesity a Matter of Personal Responsibility?

"While people surely do have some responsibility for their health, the issue of obesity says more about our society than it does about the individual."

—Mark J. Hanson, "Obesity and Responsibility."

"The only way you will lose weight permanently is to accept total responsibility for yourself and acknowledge the fact that you have the power to change, regardless of what mother nature has given you to work with."

—Tom Venuto, "Did You Inherit Fat Genes? The Truth About Biology and Body Fat."

Obesity is the fastest-growing health concern in America, and experts warn that it will only get worse. Given all the information on health and fitness today, why is obesity such a huge problem? Lifestyle choices and eating habits are often cited as primary causes of obesity. Choices made by individuals related to diet, sleeping habits, and exercise can cause obesity. But obesity is a more complex problem than that. It is also the result of the modern American way of life, in which cars, television, and fast food have taken the place of walking to shops or work, playing outside after school, and nutritious home-cooked meals. This means that often people have to go out of their way to be active and eat right. This also leaves open the question of whether obesity is entirely a matter of personal responsibility—or something more.

Individual Responsibility

Many people believe that obesity is the culmination of an individual's personal choices. People choose to buy and eat meals that are higher in fat and calories. People choose to drink large amounts of sugary soda. People choose to sit in front of their televisions, computers, game stations for hours on end. People choose to lie on the couch after dinner instead of engaging in a physical activity like walking or basketball or bicycling. John H. Sklare, a psychologist focusing on weight loss, states, "If you don't like the person looking back at you in the mirror, who do you blame? Do you own up to the damage and take the heat or do you point fingers and hold the world or someone else responsible?"[31]

> According to a California survey, 90 percent of respondents said that individuals, not the food industry, are to blame for what they eat and drink.

According to a California survey, 90 percent of respondents said that individuals, not the food industry, are to blame for what they eat and drink. Many individuals believe that taking personal responsibility for their habits and health is the first step to gaining control over obesity, while others ignore the facts of healthy eating and nutrition. Mike Adams, a holistic nutritionist, writes, "Even when most people are made aware of the health dangers of foods, they keep on eating the garbage foods anyway!"[32]

Parent Responsibility

Children learn much of what they know from the people with whom they live. Parents are the ones who teach children what to eat, when to eat it, and how much to eat. They also are in charge of how much time kids spend in front of the television and playing video games. According to diet specialist Anne Collins, "Parental behavioral patterns concerning shopping, cooking, eating and exercise have an important influence on a child's energy balance and ultimately their weight. Thus family diet and lifestyle are important contributory causes to modern child obesity."[33]

In today's always-on-the-go world, there is often not much time for preparing everyday, healthy meals. With the prevalence of processed and prepared foods, it is often easier and faster for parents to put a quick, convenient meal on the table than it is to prepare a healthy, balanced meal. The snacks parents make available are not always healthy either. However, while convenient, these ways of providing food for children do not help them avoid obesity.

> **While parents are ultimately responsible for what happens to their children, the issue of childhood obesity is not always cut and dried.**

According to the Centers for Disease Control and Prevention, between 15 and 20 percent of children in the United States are obese. While parents are ultimately responsible for what happens to their children, the issue of childhood obesity is not always cut and dried. In her book *Teenage Waistland*, Abby Ellin, a self-proclaimed former fat kid, illustrates the difficulties of this issue:

> Some parents have their own struggles with food and weight. Some waver between strategies for helping kids, and founder among the mixed messages. Some feel reluctant to structure their family's whole life around weight loss—which is what appears to be required. Others tire of trying to force a resistant kid to do something he or she doesn't want to do, creating more frustration and unhappiness in the process, upsetting and alienating their child rather than helping them.[34]

Parents often face many roadblocks when dealing with a child's weight.

School Responsibility

Many people believe that schools share some of the responsibility for obesity. According to David Foulk, professor of Health Education at Florida State University, "Lunchrooms are supposed to be cost-neutral, otherwise it comes out of the school budget. So, schools make food more appealing, providing burgers and fries and pizza."[35] Or they provide high-fat, high-sugar snacks through on-campus vending machines. Vending machines can be found in high schools and grade schools throughout the country. James O. Hill, speaking for the National Institutes of Health, says, "Many schools contain vending machines with many high energy density foods and some schools even have fast food outlets."[36]

Many schools also have exclusive contracts with soda distributors that give money back to the schools in exchange for selling only that company's products. While some schools are replacing the soda machines, in many cases the colas have been replaced with fruit juices and sports drinks that are still high in sugar. In her book *Diabesity* Francine R. Kaufmann asks, "Should students be expected to pay for any part of their education by buying things like sodas that are bad for their health?"[37]

> Sometimes physical education is the only means both older and younger students have for being involved in regular physical activity.

Sometimes physical education is the only means both older and younger students have for being involved in regular physical activity. It also provides schools with the opportunity to teach kids about the importance of physical activity. With continually rising school costs, when budget cuts are made, physical education and sports programs are often the first to be eliminated. The National Association for Sport and Physical Education (NASPE) reports that only 36 states require physical education in grade school and just 42 states require physical education during high school. Schools have an enormous impact on the lives of children and youths and can be instrumental in the obesity issue, both as a help and a hindrance.

Community Responsibility

Communities share some of the blame for obesity. The layout of many communities in the United States discourages physical activity. Most people need to use cars to get where they need to go. Grocery stores, markets, book stores, drug stores, and other retail establishments are often too far from established neighborhoods to make walking or bicycling the preferred method of transportation. While older, established communities have sidewalks, many new housing communities and subdivisions are designed without sidewalks, making it difficult to walk or ride a bicycle in the neighborhoods.

Workplaces sometimes also play a role in obesity. Stress in the workplace can be a primary cause of weight gain and other health prob-

> **On a per-calorie basis, diets composed of whole grains, fish, and fresh vegetables and fruits are far more expensive than refined grains, added sugars, and added fats.**

lems. According to the CDC, new research through the National Institute for Occupational Safety and Health (NIOSH) is being undertaken to study the links between work, obesity, and health. A NIOSH *Update*, released by the CDC, states,

> Work may promote weight gain in three ways: 1) job stress may be linked with alcohol consumption and sedentary leisure activity; 2) psychological strain could lead to modification of hormonal factors related to weight gain; and 3) long work hours, shift work, and overtime could result in fatigue, decreasing the amount of time that the individual may spend in physical activity off the job."[38]

Communities and workplaces can have an enormous impact on everyday lives and an individual's daily physical activity.

Poverty

Even if a person wants to change eating habits, buying more healthful foods is not always an option. According to Adam Drewnowski, director of the Nutritional Sciences Program at the University of Washington School of Public Health and Community Medicine, "The highest rates of obesity and type 2 diabetes are found among groups with the highest poverty rates, and the least education."[39]

One of the main connections between poverty and obesity is economic—specifically, the cost of food. Drewnowski reports that on a per-calorie basis, diets composed of whole grains, fish, and fresh vegetables and fruits are far more expensive than refined grains, added sugars, and added fats. And these costs continue to rise. According to the National Urban League, since 1985 the price of fruits and vegetables has increased 40 percent and the price of sugar and fats has decreased 14 percent.

Lean meats cost more than meats high in fat content. Ground beef is much cheaper than ground sirloin, yet ground sirloin can be up to 98 percent fat free. Francine R. Kaufmann, a medical doctor specializing in obesity and diabetes, describes a situation with one of her patients: "Her family, despite their poverty, did not go hungry. However, they were nutrition-insecure: the foods they could afford were laden with sugar and fat; fresh fruits and vegetables, lean meats, and fish were out of their reach."[40]

The American Lifestyle

American dietary habits are well known. People eat out more than they did 20 years ago, and they eat larger quantities of food. According to the U.S. Department of Agriculture, in the last four decades the amount of money spent on eating out has increased more than 20 percent. In referencing Americans, a weight-loss article from the Netherlands says, "They are replacing home cooking with fast food, dining out, and packaged foods."[41]

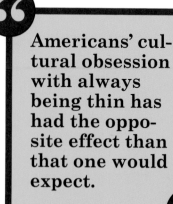

"Americans' cultural obsession with always being thin has had the opposite effect than that one would expect.

America's sedentary lifestyle is also well known. Changes in the American workplace have made the workforce much less physical than it was years ago. Many individuals start their day sitting in their cars going to work and then go from sitting all day at work to sitting in their cars getting home from work, to sitting watching television or playing video games for the evening's entertainment.

Media influence is also a big part of the obesity equation. A study done at University of California at Los Angeles has suggested that Americans' cultural obsession with always being thin has had the opposite effect than that one would expect. Instead of motivating someone to lose weight and try to deal with obesity, it actually subverts an individual's motivation to try to become healthier. Antronette Yancey, lead author of the study, is quoted as saying, "These data suggest that our society's emphasis on weight loss rather than lifestyle change may inadvertently discourage even non-obese people from adopting or maintaining the physical activity necessary for long-term good health."[42] With the continued prevalence of extremely thin role models in film, on television, and in the print media, there is little chance of the culture changing anytime soon.

Is Obesity A Matter of Personal Responsibility?

66 **Those most responsible for obesity, first and foremost, are the individuals who make poor choices about their food and diet.** 99

—Editorial Board, "Obesity Prescription: Welcome Advice, but First, Personal Responsibility," *Miami Herald*, November 3, 2007.

The *Miami Herald* is one of the largest newspapers in the United States.

66 **Ninety-nine percent of Americans believe that exercise helps preserve good health, but most feel they have to battle current culture to exercise regularly and that the government should do more to promote physical activity.** 99

—GetFit Wellness, "Current Culture Makes It Hard for People to Exercise, Four out of Five Americans Say," May 2007. www.getfitwellness.com.

GetFit Wellness provides online services and onsite motivational, training, and educational services to help individuals maintain a healthy lifestyle.

66 As individuals with free will, we can choose to grab a bag of chips, plop ourselves down in front of the TV, and slurp an extra-large soda. Or we can down a glass of water, get on our bikes and go. As individuals, we can make the better choices no matter where we live. But our environment helps shape these decisions, by making good choices easy or difficult. 99

—Francine R. Kaufman, *Diabesity*. New York: Bantam, 2005.

Kaufman is a professor of pediatrics at Keck School of Medicine at the University of Southern California.

66 When I weighed 410 pounds, I had a HUGE problem (literally!) that needed to be taken care of. . . . It was MY responsibility to take personal control of my life back by doing what I had to do to melt the fat from my body and get healthy. 99

—Jimmy Moore, "Book Claims 'Obesity Epidemic' Is a Sham," Jimmy Moore's Livin' La Vida Low-Carb Blog, November 19, 2005. http://livinlavidalocarb.blogspot.com.

Moore lost 180 pounds and is the author of *Livin' La Vida Low-Carb: My Journey from Flabby Fat to Sensationally Skinny*.

66 People are not poor by choice and they become obese primarily because they are poor. 99

—Adam Drewnowski, quoted in Ursula Snyder, "Obesity and Poverty," March/April 2004. www.medscape.com.

Drewnowski is the director of the Center for Public Health Nutrition at the University of Washington School of Public Health and Community Medicine.

66 For many women with children in poor areas the most logical food options are heavily processed foods. 99

—J. Eric Oliver, *Fat Politics*. New York: Oxford University Press, 2006.

Oliver is associate professor of political science at the University of Chicago.

66 The main problem is the extent to which manufactured, refined, and processed foods have replaced natural foods. 99

—Andrew Weil, quoted in Joan Feeney, "Technophobia Slow Cookers," *House Beautiful*, May 2007.

Weil is a well-known natural health and integrated-medicine specialist.

66 Physical education, once an important part of every child's school day, has been cut back by many schools. 99

—Mediafamily.org, "Media Use and Obesity Among Children," November 2006. www.mediafamily.org.

Mediafamily.org is run by the National Institute on Media and the Family, a research, education, and advocacy organization, focusing on positive and negative aspects of media.

66 I don't think it's right that schools are now required to limit students to lower calorie drinks. I think that I can make that decision for myself. How can anyone expect their children to make good choices on their own when they aren't teaching them, but prohibiting them from even having a decision? 99

—Katie Andrew, "From Our Readers," *Detroit Free Press*, October 15, 2007.

Andrew, a high school student, wrote this letter to the editor about her high school's new policy regarding vending machine drinks.

66 Obesity is dramatically increasing not only in American children and adults, but also in every country that has adopted similar cultural habits. 99

—Healthcentral.com, "Cultural and Emotional Causes," March 29, 2006. www.healthcentral.com.

Healthcentral.com is a network of Web sites and other media affiliates providing health information, resources, and contacts.

66 Environmental and behavioral changes brought about by economic development, modernization, and urbanization have been linked to the rise in global obesity. **99**

—American Obesity Association, "Obesity—a Global Epidemic," May 2, 2005. www.obesity.org.

The American Obesity Association focuses on public policy and obesity perceptions.

66 Instead of intervening in the array of food options available to Americans, our government ought to be working to foster a personal sense of responsibility for our health and well-being. **99**

—Radley Balko, "Are You Responsible for Your Own Weight?" *Time*, June 7, 2004.

Balko is a columnist for *FoxNews.com* and a senior editor for *Reason* magazine.

66 Imploring people to eat better and exercise more has been the default approach to obesity for years. That is a failed experiment. **99**

—Kelly Brownell and Marion Nestle, "Are You Responsible for Your Own Weight?" *Time*, June 7, 2004.

Brownell is cofounder and director of the Rudd Center for Food Policy and Obesity at Yale University and director of the Yale Center for Eating and Weight Disorders. Nestle is the Paulette Goddard Professor in New York University's Department of Nutrition, Food Studies, and Public Health. She is also the author of *Food Politics: How the Food Industry Influences Nutrition and Health*.

Facts and Illustrations

Is Obesity A Matter of Personal Responsibility?

- There are estimated to be over **71 million dieters in America**, and 70 percent try to lose weight by themselves.

- In 2008 diet soft drink sales are forecasted to reach almost **$23 billion**.

- According to the National Sleep Foundation, about **7 in 10 adults** get less than 8 hours of sleep a night on weekdays.

- From 1977 to 1996 soda consumption by teens increased by **75 percent for boys** and 40 percent for girls.

- The United States produces enough food to supply **3,800 calories a day** to every man, woman, and child.

- According to a Gallup Youth Survey, **25 percent of families** eat together at home 3 or 4 days per week, and only 28 percent of families eat together at home 7 days a week.

- According to a CDC survey, more than **50 percent of U.S. schools** offer pizza and hamburgers as a daily lunch choice.

Individual Perception of Weight in America Varies from U.S. Health Recommendations

According to an ongoing Gallup poll, 41 to 46 percent of Americans considered themselves overweight from 1990 to 2007. In contrast, the CDC reported that in 2004, 67 percent of Americans were overweight.

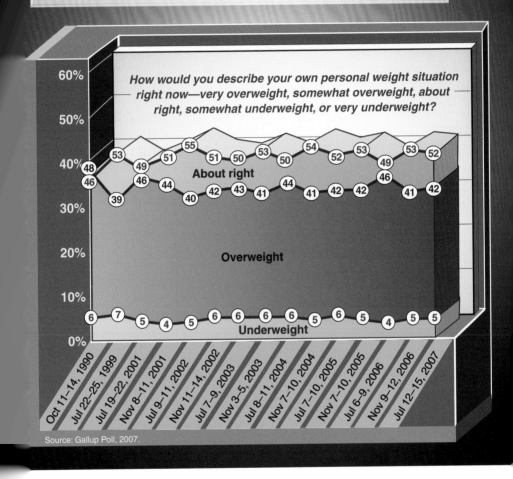

How would you describe your own personal weight situation right now—very overweight, somewhat overweight, about right, somewhat underweight, or very underweight?

Source: Gallup Poll, 2007.

• The National Association for Sport and Physical Education reports that more than **70 percent of states** require physical education for elementary school students and **65 percent** require physical education for middle school students.

Portion Sizes Increasing

In the past 5 decades portion sizes have more than doubled, tripled, and in some cases, quadrupled. Since the 1950s a single order of french fries has increased almost 300 percent. A 3-cup serving of pasta is double the size it was in 1950. Since portion sizes have increased at such a high rate, it makes it much more difficult for an individual to control the amount of food consumed.

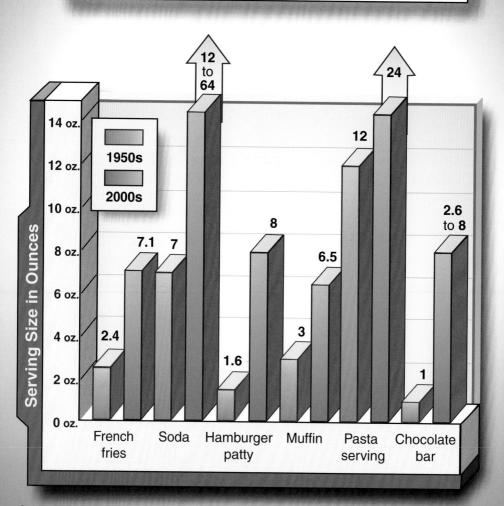

Source: www.mealsmatter.org. 2007.

Cost of Lost Work Time Due to Obesity

According to the National Institute of Diabetes & Digestive & Kidney Diseases (NIDDK), the cost of obesity-related time off has increased dramatically. Lost work productivity includes lost workday, time off for doctor visits, restricted activity time, and time off for bed-ridden days. Currently, restricted activity days are the most costly at nearly $240 million per year.

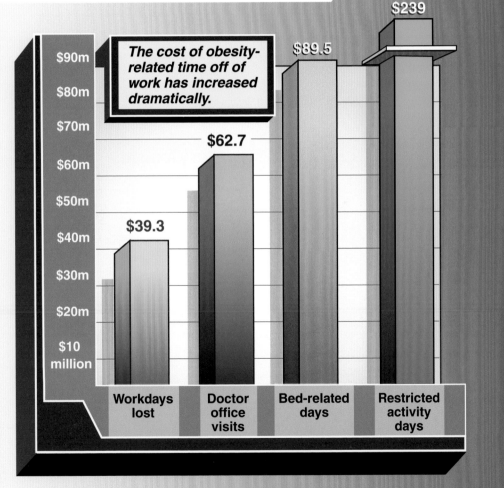

The cost of obesity-related time off of work has increased dramatically.

| | $239 |

| | $89.5 |

| | $62.7 |

| | $39.3 |

| $90m | $80m | $70m | $60m | $50m | $40m | $30m | $20m | $10 million |

| Workdays lost | Doctor office visits | Bed-related days | Restricted activity days |

Source: Weight-Control Information Network, "Statistics Related to Overweight and Obesity," www.win.niddk.nih.gov.

Number of States Requiring Physical Education in Schools

The National Association for Sport and Physical Education reports that the majority of the 50 states mandate that students take physical education classes. Over 70 percent of states require PE for elementary students and 65 percent require it for junior high students. But the No Child Left Behind Act (2001) is causing some schools to cut back on physical education time to meet the requirements for other subjects.

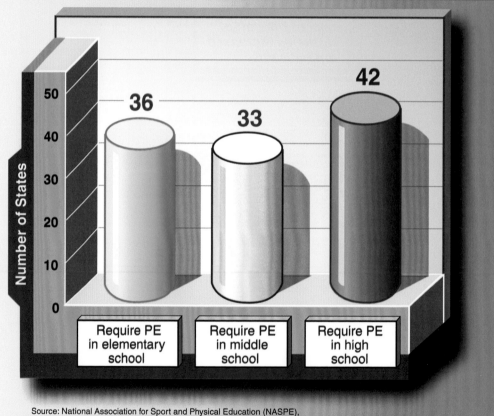

Source: National Association for Sport and Physical Education (NASPE), "Shape of the Nation Report," Executive Summary, 2006.

- According to the Center for Health and Wellbeing, **only 5 percent of** schools require physical education in grade 12.

- Nearly **30 perent** of food advertisements shown during children's programs are for fast food.

- The total cost of obesity for U.S. companies is estimated to be **$13 billion** each year.

- According to the Physicians Committee for Responsible Medicine, **less than half of 1 percent of U.S. farm bill subsidies** goes to fruit and vegetable production.

How Should Obesity Be Treated?

❝Developing permanent, healthy habits and choosing an achievable BMI goal should be the priorities.❞

—Susan Okie, *Fed Up! Winning the War Against Childhood Obesity.*

❝Treatment of obesity is generally divided into medical and surgical remedies.❞

—Louis Flancbaum, Erica Manfred, and Deborah Flancbaum, *The Doctor's Guide to Weight Loss Surgery.*

A mericans spend $50 billion a year on all kinds of weight-loss programs and treatments. Treatments for obesity fall within this broad range of weight-loss options. They include diets, drugs, surgery, and behavior-modification techniques. These treatments have a mixed rate of success for obesity. Many obesity patients find it difficult to retain the effects of dieting and weight loss. It is very common for individuals to regain lost weight after a period of successful weight loss. Medications have some success but are most successful when combined with other types of treatment. Obesity surgery can lead to significant, sustained weight loss, but it is costly and considered a last resort.

Reduced-Calorie Diets

Dieting is the single most used treatment for obesity. The most common diet is the reduced-calorie diet. This means most individuals diet by reducing the number of calories taken in while keeping the same amount of daily activity. This allows the body to burn off more calories than it is taking in. Many of these types of diets are self-administered.

If a reduced-calorie diet is followed faithfully, an individual can expect to lose approximately 20 to 40 pounds in the first 3 to 4 months. But it is not uncommon for people to gain back much of the weight they lost during the early months of a diet. *The Doctor's Guide to Weight Loss Surgery* explains, "The weight loss tends to be rapid at first but then tapers off over time, eventually reaching a plateau."[43] The plateau is reached because the body adapts to the decrease in calories.

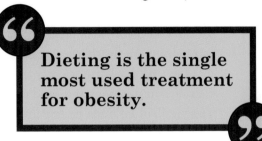

> **Dieting is the single most used treatment for obesity.**

These mechanisms that cause the body to adapt to the dieting change can lead to what has been termed "yo-yo" dieting, the process of continually gaining then losing weight.

To break the dieting plateau, most people need to make changes in levels of physical activity as well as being continually vigilant at mealtimes. These changes can include increasing physical activity, changing the amount and the types of foods eaten, and changing portion sizes (for example, eating several smaller meals throughout the day instead of three larger meals).

Behavior Modification

Behavioral therapies are often combined with diets to help obese people permanently change eating habits as well as lifestyle. Therapy programs are often conducted in groups and include lessons on self-monitoring, diet modification, restaurant eating, and motivation. Lifestyle changes can include adding more physical activity, changing the types of food and drink consumed, changing the way food is prepared, and changing the way an individual shops for food. All of these areas are key to changing behavior.

How a person changes his or her behavior is also important. Trying to make large changes all at once is a recipe for failure. A steady approach over the course of months, with small changes made at regular time intervals, is the recommended technique. Susan Okie, a family physician and medical journalist, writes, "Obesity experts emphasize that overweight kids and their families should try to make just a few small permanent changes at a time. Once they have succeeded in incorporating these changes, they can build on them by going on to the next step."[44]

If behavior is successfully changed, research has shown that obese individuals can maintain up to 60 percent of their initial weight loss. But behavior-modification treatments do not always work because few people can completely change their way of life. It is very difficult to change habits and patterns that have been ingrained for years. Louis Flancbaum, an expert on bariatric surgery, reports, "People find it hard to make a lifetime commitment and tend to revert to their old eating habits."[45] An obese individual must be extremely focused and dedicated to the goal of weight loss to change his or her behavior to the necessary degree.

Medications

When diets and behavior modification alone fail, individuals often turn to medications for help with obesity. Weight-loss medications have become increasingly popular in the last several years, with millions of prescriptions being written every year.

According to the U.S. Department of Health and Human Services Weight Control Information Network, research has shown that for long-term weight-loss success, weight-loss medications are most effective when used in conjunction with a weight program that focuses on improved eating and activity habits. Use of these medications can result in a weight loss of 5 to 22 pounds more than with nondrug treatments. This weight loss usually occurs in the first six months of treatment followed by much lower levels of weight loss or weight increases.

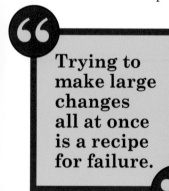

Trying to make large changes all at once is a recipe for failure.

There are two prescription medications available, but each works in a very different manner. Meridia, drug name sibutramine, works on reducing the hunger an individual experiences. It can be used long- or short-term. According to Meridia.net, "Meridia blocks the uptake of the brain chemicals (serotonin and norepinephrine) which help regulate the sense of fullness. Fullness is your signal to stop eating. Having a sense of fullness or satiety, means you may feel satisfied with less food."[46]

The other main prescription drug used to treat obesity is Xenical, drug name orlistat. Xenical works by reducing the effectiveness of the enzyme lipase. Lipase works in the small intestine to break down fat and digest the fat that is consumed in food. Xenical helps block lipase, which decreases the amount of fat and nutrients that are absorbed from food. Roche Laboratories, the maker of Xenical, states, "By working this way, Xenical helps block about one-third of the fat in the foods you eat from being absorbed by your body."[47] Blocking the absorption of fats means that an individual will absorb fewer calories with the same amount of food.

> **Use of [weight-loss] medications can result in a weight loss of 5 to 22 pounds more than with non-drug treatments.**

There are drawbacks to both. Meridia has been shown to significantly increase heart rate and blood pressure in some individuals. Individuals taking Xenical usually need a daily multivitamin because of the nonabsorption of nutrients. This medication also will cause a change in bowel habits because it works in the digestive system. Both of these medications have been shown to work best when combined with a reduced-calorie diet.

Many other medications are being investigated to see whether they will have a positive effect on obesity. Some of these drugs under scrutiny are currently being used to treat other illnesses, such as depression and epilepsy. Many times the side effects of one drug have the unintended consequence of being effective in the treatment of a different disease.

Over-the-Counter Medications and Supplements

Many over-the-counter weight-loss supplements are available today. In most magazines it is easy to find advertisements for diet pills and weight-loss supplements. The manufacturers of these products make many different claims about how they help people lose weight. Some claim to reduce calorie intake and help an individual shed excess weight without diet or exercise. Others claim to reduce stress, which in turn will reduce belly fat. Some of these claims have not been studied or proven. Many of these products promote quick and effortless weight loss, which is not usually possible for individuals struggling with obesity.

One type of supplement that is encouraged is a vitamin supplement.

While everyone does not need a vitamin supplement on a regular basis, they are often recommended for obese individuals trying to lose weight. Serious dieters often eat fewer than 1,600 calories a day, which means they are probably not getting the recommended daily allowance of certain vitamins and minerals. In this case a daily multivitamin is often recommended.

> The main difference between weight-loss supplements and FDA-approved medications is that the manufacturers of supplements do not have to prove that their products actually do what they claim.

One over-the-counter medication is approved by the Food and Drug Administration (FDA). It is called Alli (orlistat). Alli works by preventing enzymes from breaking down about one-quarter of fats eaten. GlaxoSmithKline, its maker, reports, "Because about a quarter of the fat can't be absorbed, it passes out of your body instead of turning into calories."[48] This medication is designed to work with a weight-loss plan.

The main difference between weight-loss supplements and FDA-approved medications is that the manufacturers of supplements do not have to prove that their products actually do what they claim. In *Time* magazine, Dr. Sanjay Gupta reports, "In more than two-thirds of cases, the preparations have never been clinically proved to be effective for those uses."[49] To get FDA approval, nonprescription or over-the-counter medications must have clinical-trial evidence that they work. Each year more and more weight-loss products appear on the American market and, if used, should be evaluated by a doctor for potential risks and side effects. These products can sometimes be used in conjunction with one another for more effectiveness, but most are more effective when combined with a reduced-calorie diet and increased physical activity.

Cosmetic Surgery and More

One of the more radical obesity treatments an individual can undergo is surgery. Several types of surgery are used to treat obesity, and each one has advantages and disadvantages. Cosmetic surgery is used for some obesity patients. These surgical treatments include liposuction and abdomino-plasty. Abdominoplasty, one of the most common cosmetic surgeries, is also known as a "tummy tuck." Laparoscopy is used to remove excess skin and fat deposits from the abdomen. Often, obese individuals can develop abdominal hernias. Many times, when surgery is performed to correct the hernia, obese patients have abdominoplasty at the same time. Complications with this surgery can include poor healing, resulting in large scars and, in some cases, infections and blood clots.

Liposuction is the removal of fat deposits from beneath the skin. The results from this type of surgical procedure are immediate but do not affect an individual's overall long-term weight. If an individual has liposuction but makes no changes in lifestyle or eating habits, excess fat will build up in other places. The Web site Liposuction.com reports, "Unrealistic expectations are the most frequent source of disappointing liposuction results."[50] Another main drawback is the occurrence of depressions and irregularities in the skin following a procedure.

One of the newest surgery-based obesity treatments is the installation of an implantable gastric stimulator (IGS). This device works much like a cardiac pacemaker. *Newsweek* reports, "The pacemaker-like device is implanted in the abdominal wall and attached through two electrodes to the stomach muscle. It affects the biochemistry of the gut, making you feel fuller faster."[51] This feeling of fullness helps control the amount of food an individual will actually eat, which will in turn affect his or her overall weight.

> **Gastric banding surgery reduces the size of the stomach's volume, usually resulting in long-term weight loss.**

Bariatric Surgery

Bariatric surgery is the most radical obesity treatment. This type of surgery involves major surgical adjustments to an individual's digestive system. The two most common bariatric procedures that lead to significant weight loss are gastric banding and gastric bypass.

Gastric banding surgery reduces the size of the stomach's volume, usually resulting in long-term weight loss. Two types of gastric banding are the most popular: adjustable gastric banding and vertical gastric banding. In vertical gastric banding, the stomach is made smaller by a vertical line of staples, and a band is placed to allow a slower emptying of the stomach. With adjustable gastric banding, an adjustable band is placed around the upper section of the stomach to limit food intake. The band can be inflated or deflated to make the stomach volume larger or smaller. Susan Okie, author of *Fed Up!* writes, "In addition to reducing stomach capacity, the procedures seem to reduce appetite, probably by altering the levels of various chemical messengers produced in the stomach and intestinal tract that influence perceptions of hunger and satiety."[52]

Gastric bypass surgery, or gastroplasty, actually changes the routing of the digestive system. This greatly reduces the body's ability to take in and process vitamins and other nutrients from food, usually causing quick weight loss. There are several types of this kind of obesity surgery. Roux-en-Y surgery closes off most of the stomach and reroutes it to the middle section of the small intestine. This not only makes the stomach much smaller, it bypasses the first part of the small intestine and reduces the amount of materials and nutrients that can be absorbed.

Regarding related complications, obesity and diabetes expert Francine R. Kaufmann states, "An estimated 10 to 20 percent of those who undergo bariatric surgery subsequently require additional surgery to correct problems, such as abdominal hernias. Many patients develop gallstones, a common consequence of rapid weight loss."[53]

Because of possible complications, obesity surgery is often the last resort of many obese individuals. Denise Rasley underwent bariatric surgery in 1998 and lost 180 pounds. She states, "After surgery it was like I started my life all over again."[54]

Primary Source Quotes*

How Should Obesity Be Treated?

66 There's no doubt that a properly informed individual can take control over their health outcome and utterly avoid obesity and chronic disease, especially if they engage in optimum nutrition, take various nutritional supplements and add superfoods to their diets. 99

—Mike Adams, "Is Obesity a Choice or a Disease?" *NewsTarget.com*, July 19, 2004. www.newstarget.com.

Adams is a holistic nutritionist.

66 The purpose of behavior modification therapy in obese people is to help change behaviors that contribute to obesity and initiate new dietary and physical activity behaviors that are needed to lose weight. 99

—Erica Lesperance, "Treatment of Childhood Obesity: Behavior Modification Therapy," January 17, 2007. www.thedietchannel.com.

Lesperance is a registered dietician specializing in metabolic nutrition.

Bracketed quotes indicate conflicting positions.

* Editor's Note: While the definition of a primary source can be narrowly or broadly defined, for the purposes of Compact Research, a primary source consists of: 1) results of original research presented by an organization or researcher; 2) eyewitness accounts of events, personal experience, or work experience; 3) first-person editorials offering pundits' opinions; 4) government officials presenting political plans and/or policies; 5) representatives of organizations presenting testimony or policy.

"When you really, really study the numbers critically closely, there really isn't this big spike in fatness, in overweight or obesity that is both the prevailing wisdom and also the rationale for the government doing all kinds of things to turn around this tide."

—Patrick Basham, "Counterpoint: The Obesity Myth," ABC Radio National, April 16, 2007.

Basham is coauthor of *Diet Nation* and director of the Democracy Institute in Washington, D.C.

"The best advice is to avoid weight loss supplements, which generally do not work and may be dangerous."

—Health A to Z, "Obesity Treatments," June 2007. www.healthatoz.com.

Health A to Z is a health and medical resource developed by health-care professionals.

"From thyroid treatments in the early twentieth century to methamphetamines in the 1950s to liquid protein diets of the 1980s to fen-phen in the 1990s, American doctors have promoted a host of dangerous drugs and treatments for people wanting to be thin."

—J. Eric Oliver, *Fat Politics: The Real Story Behind America's Obesity Epidemic.* New York: Oxford University Press, 2006.

Oliver is associate professor of political science at the University of Chicago.

"Weight loss surgery takes people who are a lot overweight and makes them a lot less overweight."

—Louis Flancbaum, Erica Manfred, and Deborah Flancbaum, *The Doctor's Guide to Weight Loss Surgery.* New York: Bantam.

Flancbaum is a general surgeon and a specialist in bariatric surgery. Manfred is a writer and medical journalist. Flancbaum is a writer.

---

66 For anybody who thinks this is a magic bullet, you do this and it's done. You're making a mistake. It's not. **99**

—Al Roker, "Weighing the Risks: Al's Update," *Dateline NBC*, November 5, 2004. www.msnbc.msn.com.

Roker is the weather anchor on NBC's *Today* show and is a features reporter for NBC News. Roker underwent gastric bypass surgery in 2002.

66 This surgery has changed my life and is the best thing that I have ever done for myself. After my long 35-year struggle with obesity, I feel for the first time, that I am a regular-sized person. **99**

—Carolyn Williamson, "Obesity Control Center Patient Testimonial," 2007. www.obesitycontrolcenter.com.

Williamson lost more than 100 pounds after having Lap Band surgery.

66 A diet that is individually planned to help create a deficit of 500 to 1,000 kcal/day should be an integral part of any program aimed at achieving a weight loss of 1 to 2 pounds per week. **99**

—National Heart Lung and Blood Institute, Obesity Education Initiative, "Aim for a Healthy Weight: Key Recommendations," 2007. www.nhlbi.nih.gov.

The National Heart Lung and Blood Institute is part of the National Institutes of Health and focuses on causes, prevention, diagnosis, and treatment of heart, blood vessel, lung, and blood diseases, as well as sleep disorders.

66 A statistic frequently used about obesity treatment is that 95 percent of people who lose weight gain it all back. That statistic, based on a small study from 1959, is no longer valid. Much has changed in the way of obesity treatment since then. **99**

—American Obesity Association, "AOA Fact Sheets: Obesity Treatment," May 2, 2005. www.obesity1.tempdomainname.com.

The American Obesity Association is an advocacy organization offering obesity information and focusing on public policy related to obesity.

Facts and Illustrations

How Should Obesity Be Treated?

- According to the *Journal News*, more than **1 million children** have used personal trainers to lose weight, improve their fitness level, or improve their sports skills. This amounts to 17 percent of the 6.3 million people who used personal trainers.

- Abbott Laboratories reports approximately **14 million people** in more than 75 countries have used Meridia (sibutramine) to treat obesity since it was introduced in 1997.

- Roche Laboratories states that in clinical studies, **after 52 weeks** those patients using Xenical along with a reduced-calorie diet lost an average of twice as much weight as the patients using diet alone.

- *Time* magazine reports that the sale of herbal supplements was **$22.3 billion** in 2006.

- According to the American Society of Plastic Surgeons, in 2006 more than **300,000 liposuction procedures** were performed in the United States.

- Ads for high-fat and high-salt foods have increased **more than 100 percent** since the 1980s.

- According to the CDC, roughly **25 percent of adults** in the United States eat the recommended five or more servings of fruit and vegetables every day.

Weight-Loss Market in Dollars

The U.S. weight-loss market has skyrocketed in the past 4 years, increasing more than $15 billion from 2002–2006. Marketdata Enterprises estimates that by 2010 the market will increase to more than $68 billion.

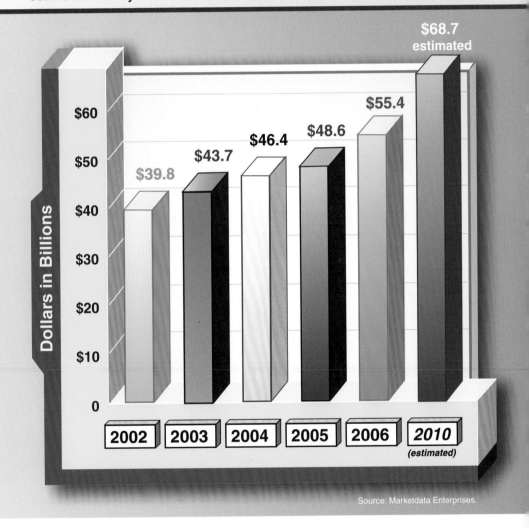

Source: Marketdata Enterprises.

- The American Society for Bariatric Surgery reports a complication **rate of 5 percent** and a mortality rate of 0.5 percent in Roux-en-Y bypass patients in 2004.

The Risks of Obesity Surgery Increase with Age

As age increases, the risk of mortality from obesity surgery also rises slightly. For men, the risk stays under 10 percent until ages 65–74. At that age the rate rises to a little over 10 percent. For women, the mortality rate is less than 10 percent through age 74. For both sexes, at age 75 and older, the risk increases dramatically to 40 percent for women and more than 50 percent for men.

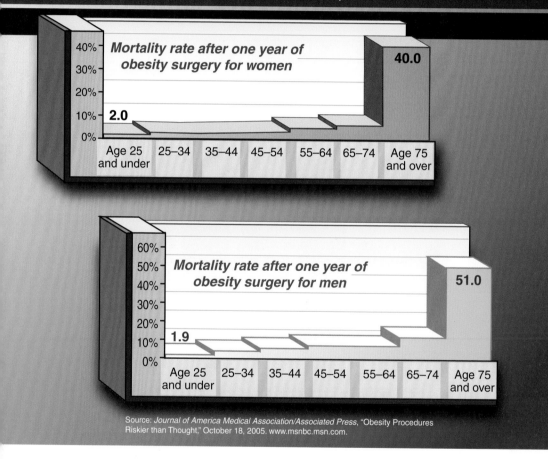

Mortality rate after one year of obesity surgery for women

Age 25 and under	25–34	35–44	45–54	55–64	65–74	Age 75 and over
2.0						40.0

Mortality rate after one year of obesity surgery for men

Age 25 and under	25–34	35–44	45–54	55–64	65–74	Age 75 and over
1.9						51.0

Source: *Journal of America Medical Association/Associated Press*, "Obesity Procedures Riskier than Thought," October 18, 2005. www.msnbc.msn.com.

- Marketdata Enterprises forecasts that the commercial chain weight-loss center market will grow to **$2.6 billion** in 2008.

- The total weight-loss market is expected to be nearly **$61 billion** by 2008, according to Marketdata Enterprises.

- According to VIMO, a health-care cost comparison Web site, the average list price for obesity treatment surgical procedures is **$41,100**; the average negotiated price is $15,400.

- The average American woman is **13 pounds heavier** now than in 1970; the average American man is 7 pounds heavier.

Typical Bariatric Surgery Characteristics

The Bariatric Surgery Registry reports that most patients having obesity surgery have the charted characteristics. Seventy-five percent of surgery patients have a BMI of 40 or more, categorizing them as extremely obese.

Average weight at time of surgery	**279.4 pounds**
Average BMI at time of surgery	46
% of surgery patients with BMI of 35 to 39.99	19.7%
% of surgery patients with BMI of at least 40	76.1%

Source: Obesity in America, www.obesityinamerica.org.

- According to Trust for America's Health, **obesity rates rose** in 31 states in 2006, rose in 22 states for the second straight year, and dropped in no state.

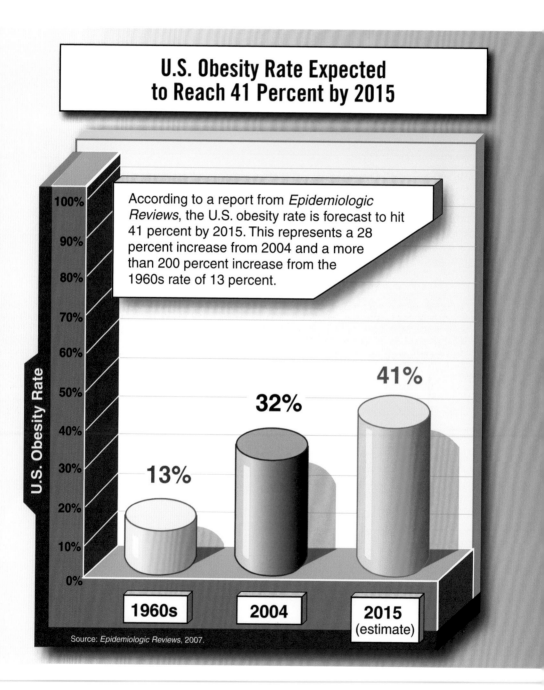

U.S. Obesity Rate Expected to Reach 41 Percent by 2015

According to a report from *Epidemiologic Reviews*, the U.S. obesity rate is forecast to hit 41 percent by 2015. This represents a 28 percent increase from 2004 and a more than 200 percent increase from the 1960s rate of 13 percent.

U.S. Obesity Rate

100%
90%
80%
70%
60%
50%
40%
30%
20%
10%
0%

13% — 1960s
32% — 2004
41% — 2015 (estimate)

Source: *Epidemiologic Reviews*, 2007.

Key People and Advocacy Groups

Louis J. Aronne: Aronne is an obesity specialist. He has authored more than 40 book chapters and papers on the subject of obesity and is Clinical Professor of Medicine at Cornell University's Weill Medical College.

Kelly Brownell: Brownell, a Yale psychologist, is director of the Yale Center for Eating and Weight Disorders. He is the author of *Food Fight* and has suggested a tax on soft drinks and junk food.

Paul F. Campos: Campos is a professor at the University of Colorado School of Law and author of *The Obesity Myth: Why America's Obesession with Weight Is Hazardous to Your Health*. With this book he challenges the idea that there is an obesity epidemic.

Center for Science in the Public Interest: CSPI is a nutrition and health consumer advocacy organization providing information to government policy makers and the public. CSPI also conducts research on food, alcohol, and health issues.

Chevy Chase: Chase is an actor and, with his wife Jayni, founder of the Center for Environmental Education Online. He testified before Congress regarding obesity in May 2007.

Leonard Epstein: Epstein is the head of Stanford University's Pediatric Weight Control Program. He pioneered the use of behavioral modification therapy along with diet and exercise programs to treat obesity in children.

James O. Hill: Hill is director of the Center for Human Nutrition at the University of Colorado Health Sciences Center. He is a leading authority on obesity and weight management.

Marion Nestle: Nestle is the Paulette Goddard Professor in New York University's Department of Nutrition, Food Studies, and Public Health. Nestle concentrates her nutrition research on social factors that influence how and why people choose certain foods. She is the author of *What to Eat, Safe Food,* and *Food Politics.*

MeMe Roth: Roth is president and founder of the advocacy group National Action Against Obesity (NAAO). She has appeared on various national television news programs stressing the dangers of obesity.

Shaping America's Health: Association for Weight Management and Obesity Prevention: Founded by the American Diabetes Association, this organization focuses on the health consequences of obesity and being overweight. It provides obesity and health information and support to families, individuals, communities, and health professionals.

Morgan Spurlock: Spurlock is an independent documentary filmmaker, TV producer, and screenwriter. He is best known for his documentary *Super Size Me,* which brought national attention to the obesity issue.

Pattie Thomas: Thomas is the coauthor of *Taking Up Space: How Eating Well and Exercising Regularly Changed My Life*. As a medical sociologist, Thomas focuses on the physical, emotional, and economic costs of obesity.

Marilyn Wann: Wann is the founder of the magazine *Fat!So?* and author of a book of the same title. She is the Activism Chair of the Board of Directors of the National Association to Advance Fat Acceptance and a key individual in the fat activism (or acceptance) movement.

Chronology

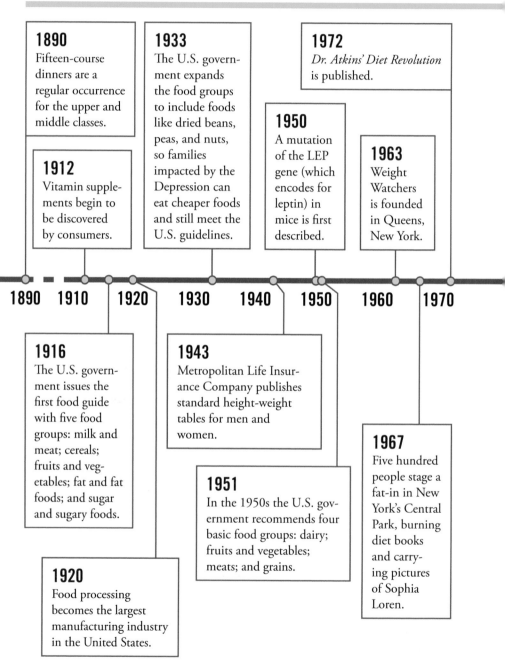

1890
Fifteen-course dinners are a regular occurrence for the upper and middle classes.

1912
Vitamin supplements begin to be discovered by consumers.

1933
The U.S. government expands the food groups to include foods like dried beans, peas, and nuts, so families impacted by the Depression can eat cheaper foods and still meet the U.S. guidelines.

1972
Dr. Atkins' Diet Revolution is published.

1950
A mutation of the LEP gene (which encodes for leptin) in mice is first described.

1963
Weight Watchers is founded in Queens, New York.

1890 1910 1920 1930 1940 1950 1960 1970

1916
The U.S. government issues the first food guide with five food groups: milk and meat; cereals; fruits and vegetables; fat and fat foods; and sugar and sugary foods.

1943
Metropolitan Life Insurance Company publishes standard height-weight tables for men and women.

1951
In the 1950s the U.S. government recommends four basic food groups: dairy; fruits and vegetables; meats; and grains.

1967
Five hundred people stage a fat-in in New York's Central Park, burning diet books and carrying pictures of Sophia Loren.

1920
Food processing becomes the largest manufacturing industry in the United States.

Chronology

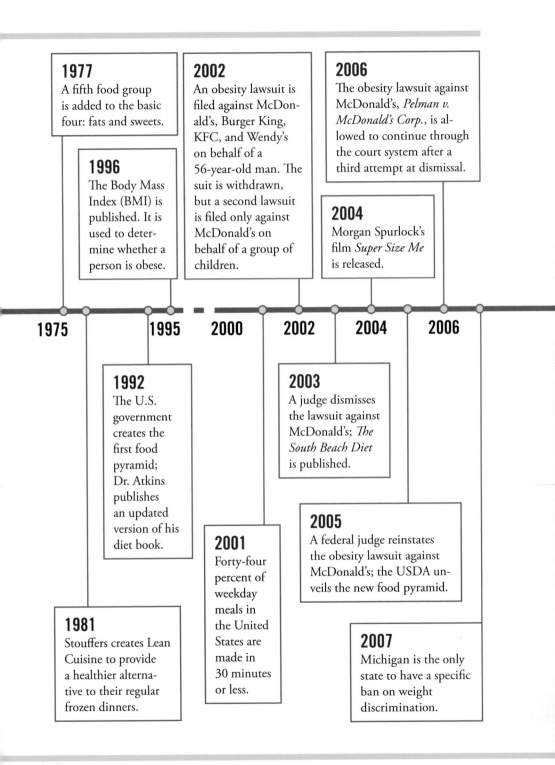

1977
A fifth food group is added to the basic four: fats and sweets.

1996
The Body Mass Index (BMI) is published. It is used to determine whether a person is obese.

2002
An obesity lawsuit is filed against McDonald's, Burger King, KFC, and Wendy's on behalf of a 56-year-old man. The suit is withdrawn, but a second lawsuit is filed only against McDonald's on behalf of a group of children.

2006
The obesity lawsuit against McDonald's, *Pelman v. McDonald's Corp.*, is allowed to continue through the court system after a third attempt at dismissal.

2004
Morgan Spurlock's film *Super Size Me* is released.

1975   1995   2000   2002   2004   2006

1992
The U.S. government creates the first food pyramid; Dr. Atkins publishes an updated version of his diet book.

2003
A judge dismisses the lawsuit against McDonald's; *The South Beach Diet* is published.

2001
Forty-four percent of weekday meals in the United States are made in 30 minutes or less.

2005
A federal judge reinstates the obesity lawsuit against McDonald's; the USDA unveils the new food pyramid.

1981
Stouffers creates Lean Cuisine to provide a healthier alternative to their regular frozen dinners.

2007
Michigan is the only state to have a specific ban on weight discrimination.

Related Organizations

Related Organizations

American Obesity Association (AOA)

1250 24th St. NW, Ste. 300

Washington, DC 20037

phone: (202) 776-7711 • fax: (202) 776-7712

e-mail: executive@obesity.org

Web site: www.obesity1.tempdomainname.com

The AOA is an organization concentrating on changing public policy and perceptions regarding obesity. Its Web site contains information on many different areas of obesity, including fact sheets, advocacy updates, consumer alerts, and research information.

The Center for Consumer Freedom

PO Box 34557

Washington, DC 20043

phone: (202) 463-7112

Web site: www.consumerfreedom.com

This consumer advocacy group consisting of restaurants, food companies, and consumers focuses on personal responsibility and protecting consumer choice in regard to food and drink choices. Its Web site contains information on the obesity debate and the obesity myth, op-eds, a news archive, and more.

Centers for Disease Control and Prevention (CDC)

1600 Clifton Rd.

Atlanta, GA 30333

phone: (404) 639-3311

Web site: www.cdc.gov

The CDC is part of the U.S. Department of Health and Human Services and focuses on disease prevention and research. The organization disseminates large amounts of information on chronic diseases and health conditions. Its Web site contains information on obesity causes, consequences, treatments, FAQs, and information on obesity organizations.

Medical News Today

PO Box 193

Bexhill-on-Sea

East Sussex, TN40 9BA, United Kingdom

e-mail: editors@medicalnewstoday.com

Web site: www.medicalnewstoday.com

This medical news and information Web site publishes the latest obesity headlines and news stories.

National Action Against Obesity (NAAO)

e-mail: info@actionagainstobesity.com

Web site: www.actionagainstobesity.com

This obesity organization focuses on removing junk food from the food supply and barring junk food from schools. The organization largely relies on parental involvement and action. Its Web site contains press releases and an extensive listing of friends-and-advocates links.

National Association to Advance Fat Acceptance (NAAFA)

PO Box 22510

Oakland, CA 94609

phone: (916) 558-6880

e-mail: webmaster@naafa.org • Web site: www.naafa.org

NAAFA works to improve the quality of life and eliminate discrimination for overweight and obese individuals. Its Web site contains information brochures on a variety of subjects, local chapter information, events information, and legal information through the Persons with Disabilities Law Center.

National Institutes of Health (NIH)

9000 Rockville Pike

Bethesda, MD 20892

phone: (301) 496-4000

e-mail: nihinfo@od.nih.gov • Web site: www.nih.gov

The NIH conducts and supports research on human diseases and disorders, human growth and development, and biological concerns of environmental contaminants. It also conducts programs to collect, disseminate, and exchange information on these subjects. The NIH Web site contains a large amount of information on many diseases and disorders, including obesity and related conditions.

North American Association for the Study of Obesity: the Obesity Society

8630 Tenton St., Ste. 918

Silver Spring, MD 20910

phone: (301) 563-6526 • fax: (301) 563-6595

e-mail: webmaster@naaso.org • Web site: www.naaso.org

NAASO stands for the North American Association for the Study of Obesity. This organization focuses on encouraging research into the causes and treatments of obesity. The Web site contains general obesity information, case study information, obesity management information, and position statements.

ObesityinAmerica.org

phone: (301) 941-0200

e-mail: media@endo-society.org

ObesityinAmerica.org is a joint program of the Endocrine Society (www.endo-society.org) and the Hormone Foundation (www.hormone.org), an affiliate of the Endocrine Society. The Endocrine Society focuses on research, education, and medical practice of endocrinology and metabolism, including the study of obesity. Its Web site contains a variety of obesity information, including obesity basics, trends, initiatives, and resources.

U.S. Department of Agriculture (USDA)

1400 Independence Ave. SW

Washington, DC 20250

Web site: www.usda.gov

The USDA covers all aspects of farming, agriculture, nutrition, and food for the United States. The Food & Nutrition section of its Web site contains information on obesity prevention, meal planning, nutrition programs, food safety fact sheets, and MyPyramid, which includes individualized nutrition planning. The Web site also contains a listing of directories for the entire department, a general inquiry and feedback form, and an "ask an expert" form.

Weight-Control Information Network (WIN)

1 WIN Way

Bethesda, MD 20892-3665

phone: (877) 946-4627 • fax: (202) 828-1028

e-mail: win@info.niddk.nih.gov • Web site: www.win.niddk.nih.gov

WIN is an information service of the National Institute of Diabetes and Digestive and Kidney Diseases (NIDDK), part of the National Institutes of Health (NIH). WIN provides science-based information and resources on weight control, obesity, physical activity, and nutritional issues to the public, media, health professionals, and Congress. Its Web site contains many publications regarding these issues.

For Further Research

Books

American Medical Association, *Assessment and Management of Adult Obesity*. Atlanta, GA: American Medical Association, 2003.

Greg Critser, *Fatland: How Americans Became the Fattest People in the World*. Boston: Houghton Mifflin, 2003.

Marie Demers, *Walk for Your Life! Restoring Neighborhood Walkways to Enhance Community Life, Improve Street Safety, and Reduce Obesity*. Ridgefield, CT: Vital Health, 2005.

Abby Ellin, *Teenage Waistland: A Former Fat Kid Weighs in on Living Large, Losing Weight, and How Parents Can (and Can't) Help*. New York: Public Affairs, 2005.

Jeanne Albronda Heaton and Claudia J. Strauss, *Talking to Eating Disorders: Simple Ways to Support Someone with Anorexia, Bulimia, Binge Eating, or Body Image Issues*. New York: New American Library, 2005.

Francine R. Kaufman, *Diabesity: The Obesity-Diabetes Epidemic That Threatens America—and What We Must Do to Stop It*. New York: Bantam, 2005.

David M. Nathan and Linda M. Delahanty, *Beating Diabetes*. New York: McGraw Hill, 2005.

Marion Nestle, *Food Politics: How the Food Industry Influences Nutrition and Health*. Berkeley and Los Angeles: University of California Press, 2003.

Byron J. Richards and Mary Guignon Richards, *Mastering Leptin: The Leptin Diet, Solving Obesity and Preventing Disease*. 2nd ed. Minneapolis: Wellness Resources, 2004.

Eric Schlosser, *Fast Food Nation*. Boston: Houghton Mifflin, 2001.

William Sears, Martha Sears, James Sears, and Robert Sears, *The Healthiest Kid in the Neighborhood*. New York: Little, Brown, 2006.

Morgan Spurlock, *Don't Eat This Book: Fast Food and the Supersizing of America*. New York: Putnam, 2005.

Kimberly A. Tessmer, Meghan Beecher, and Shelly Hagan, *Conquering Childhood Obesity for Dummies*. Hoboken, NJ: Wiley, 2006.

Pattie Thomas and Carl Wilkerson, *Taking Up Space: How Eating Well and Exercising Regularly Changed My Life*. Nashville, TN: PearlSong, 2005.

Periodicals

Jeffrey S. Flier and Eleftheria Maratos-Flier, "What Fuels Fat," *Scientific American*, September 2007.

Sanjay Gupta, "Buyer Beware," *Time*, June 4, 2007.

Kerry Hannon, "Workout Vacations," *U.S. News & World Report*, June 4, 2007.

Mike Hughlett, "Government Fighting to Get Between You and Your Cheeseburger," *Chicago Tribune*, September 12, 2007.

Jeffrey Kluger, "The Science of Appetite," *Time*, June 11, 2007.

———, "Why We Eat," *Time*, June 7, 2004.

Kim Kozlowski, "Diet Pill: Big Hopes for Smaller Sizes," *Detroit News*, June 12, 2007.

Michael D. Lemonick, "How We Grew So Big," *Time*, June 7, 2004.

———, "The Science of Addiction," *Time*, July 16, 2007.

Jeremy Manier, "Obesity May Cut U.S. Life Spans, Study Says," *Chicago Tribune*, March 17, 2005.

Eric Nagourney, "Patterns: Children's Ads on TV Push Sugar and Fat," *New York Times*, September 11, 2007.

Marion Nestle, "Eating Made Simple," *Scientific American*, September 2007.

Amy Paturel, "Overstuffed," *Better Homes and Gardens*, September 2007.

Paul Raeburn, "Can Fat Be Fit?" *Scientific American*, September 2007.

Lynn Schnurnberger, "How to Raise a Heathy Eater," *Parade*, August 26, 2007.

Edie Shaw-Ewald, "Midnight Mass," *Better Homes and Gardens*, August 2007.

Karen Tumulty, "The Politics of Fat," *Time*, March 27, 2006.

Anne Underwood and Jerry Adler, "What You Don't Know About Fat," *Newsweek*, August 23, 2004.

Internet Sources

American Cancer Society, "Controlling Portion Sizes," October 2, 2006. www.cancer.org.

Sarah Arnquist, "How to Beat Obesity," *Gelf Magazine*, October 3, 2005. www.gelfmagazine.com.

Associated Press, "Study: Obesity Surgery Riskier than Thought," October 19, 2005. www.usatoday.com.

Center for Consumer Freedom, "An Epidemic of Obesity Myths," June 2, 2004. www.consumerfreedom.com.

The Future of Children, "Childhood Obesity," Spring 2006. www.futureofchildren.org.

Samantha Henig, "Battle of the Binge," February 2, 2007. www.msnbc.msn.com/id/16945310/site/newsweek.

International Food Information Council, "Questions and Answers About Fructose," April 2005. http://ific.org.

National Heart Lung and Blood Institute, "Portion Distortion Quiz." http://hp2010.nhlbihin.net/portion.

Office of the Surgeon General, "Overweight and Obesity: Health Consequences," January 11, 2007. www.surgeongeneral.gov/topics/obesity/calltoaction.

St. Vincent Health, "What Causes Obesity?" 2006. www.stvincent.org.

U.S. Department of Health and Human Services, "Economic Consequences," January 11, 2007. www.surgeongeneral.gov/topics/obesity.

Julie Watson, "Eat to Live: Obesity's Officially Genetic!" April 13, 2007. www.sciencedaily.com.

Web Sites

Anne Collins (www.annecollins.com). This e-diet and weight management site offers a large amount of obesity information, including general background, health consequences, children and teen information, surgical treatments, and other topics.

MedicineNet.com (www.medicinenet.com). This medical information site provides many articles on obesity and related topics.

Medline Plus (www.nlm.nih.gov). This medical information site is a service of the U.S. National Library of Medicine. The site offers a broad range of information on various aspects of obesity, including basic information, coping strategies, research information, reference links, and other related issues.

NewsTarget.com (www.newstarget.com). This natural health education and information site offers articles on obesity and related topics. The site can be critical of the conventional medical establishment.

Office of the Surgeon General: "The Surgeon General's Call to Action to Prevent and Decrease Overweight and Obesity." (www. surgeongeneral.gov). This U.S. government site offers fact sheets covering many aspects of obesity, including general information, health consequences, weight advice, treatments, children and teens, and others. The site also has links to other government resources regarding obesity.

ScienceDaily **(www.sciencedaily.com).** This science site offers news and articles on science, technology, medicine, and current research regarding these topics. The site also has many links to other related information.

World Health Organization (www.who.int/topics/obesity/en). This site offers a wider perspective on obesity, including basic global obesity information, fact sheets, and regional information. It also covers nutrition, diet and exercise, and other topics.

Source Notes

Overview

1. Quoted in Mediawise.org, "Media Use and Obesity Among Children," November 2006. www.mediafamily.org.

2. Anne Collins, "Causes of Obesity," May 2007. www.annecollins.com.

3. Julia Watson, "Eat to Live: Obesity's Officially Genetic!" *ScienceDaily*, April 13, 2007. www.sciencedaily.com.

4. Stephen O'Rahilly, "Causes of Obesity," May 2007. www.annecollins.com.

5. George A. Bray, "Etiology and Natural History of Obesity," 2007. www.patients.uptodate.com.

6. Centers for Disease Control and Prevention, "About BMI for Adults," May 22, 2007. www.cdc.gov.

7. Centers for Disease Control and Prevention, "About BMI for Children and Teens," May 22, 2007 www.cdc.gov.

8. Grocery Manufacturers Association, "Consumers Say Responsibility for Obesity Lies with Individuals," March 26, 2003. www.gmabrands.com.

9. Quoted in Kim Severson, "Turning the Tables on America's Diet," *San Francisco Chronicle*, August 12, 2004. www.sfgate.com.

10. U.S. Department of Agriculture, "Steps to a Healthier You," 2007. www.mypyramid.gov.

11. William Hunter, *Medications and Surgeries for Weight Loss: When Dieting Isn't Enough.* Philadelphia: Mason Crest, 2006, p. 22.

12. Michael Childress, "Future Obesity and Smoking Rates," Kentucky Long Term Policy Research Center *Policy Notes*, no. 20, March 2006, p. 2.

What Are the Causes of Obesity?

13. National Center for Biotechnology Information, "Obesity," July 3, 2007. www.ncbi.nlm.nih.gov.

14. Centers for Disease Control and Prevention, "Overweight and Obesity: An Overview," May 22, 2007. www.cdc.gov.

15. Rhode Island Department of Health, "Initiative for a Healthy Weight: The Obesity Epidemic, Environmental Factors That Contribute to Obesity," 2007. www.health.state.ri.us.

16. Kristin Leutwyler Ozelli, "This Is Your Brain on Food," *Scientific American*, vol. 297, no. 3, September 2007, p. 85.

17. Quoted in Marilynn Larkin, "The Lack of Willpower," *New York Times*, August 29, 2007. www.nytimes.com.

18. St. Vincent Health, "What Causes Obesity?" 2006. www.stvincent.org.

19. Cleveland Clinic, "Causes of Obesity Involve Many Factors," 2007. http://cms.clevelandclinic.org.

20. *ScienceDaily*, "Obesity Causes Breakdown in System Which Regulates Appetite and Weight," March 8, 2007. www.sciencedaily.com.

21. Endocrine and Metabolic Diseases Information Service, "Cushing's Syndrome," NIH Publication No. 02-3007, June 2002, p. 1.

How Can Obesity Be Prevented?

22. United States Department of Agriculture, "Steps to a Healthier Weight," 2007. www.mypyramid.gov.

23. Centers for Disease Control and Pre-

vention, "Overweight and Obesity: An Overview."

24. National Sleep Foundation, "Myths—and Facts—About Sleep," 2007. www.sleepfoundation.org.

25. Anne Harding, "More Family Meals May Help Keep Kids Slim," Reuters Health, January 10, 2007. www.shapingamericashealth.org.

26. Quoted in Harding, "More Family Meals May Help Keep Kids Slim."

27. Reuters Health, "Kids May Pack on Pounds During the Summer," February 28, 2007. www.shapingamericas health.org.

28. Centers for Disease Control and Prevention, "Obesity and Overweight: State Based Programs," May 22, 2007. www.cdc.gov.

29. Charlene Rennick, "Reducing Obesity in the Workplace," *American Chronicle*, May 15, 2007. www.americanchronicle. com.

30. Mike Adams, "Employers Must Take On Some Responsibility for Employees' Health in Order to Prevent Obesity and Chronic Disease," *NewsTarget*, August 5, 2004. www.newstarget.com.

Is Obesity a Matter of Personal Responsibility?

31. John H. Sklare, "Personal Responsibility for Obesity Prevention," *LifeScript*, December 5, 2005. www.lifescript.com.

32. Mike Adams, "Is Obesity a Choice or a Disease?" *NewsTarget*, July 19, 2004. www.newstarget.com.

33. Collins, "Causes of Obesity."

34. Abby Ellin, *Teenage Waistland*. New York: Public Affairs, p. xxxvi.

35. Quoted in Stephen Spotswood, "NIH Highlights Link Between Obesity and Environment," *US Medicine*, July

2004. www.usmedicine.com.

36. James O. Hill, "Addressing the Environment to Reduce Obesity," National Institutes of Health. www.niehs.nih. gov.

37. Francine Kaufman, *Diabesity*. New York: Bantam, 2005, p. 237.

38. Centers for Disease Control and Prevention, National Institute for Occupational Safety and Health, "Research Challenges in Work, Obesity, and Health Examined by NIOSH Scientists, Colleague in Paper," April 11, 2007. www.cdc.gov.

39. Quoted in Craig Degginger, "USDA Study to Address Obesity and Poverty," University of Washington Office of News and Information, June 22, 2004. http://uwnews.washington.edu.

40. Kaufman, *Diabesity*, p. 207.

41. PreVital, "What Are the Cultural and Emotional Causes of Obesity?" 2006. www.prevital.nl.

42. Quoted in UCLA, "Focus on Weight Undermines Motivation for Healthy Lifestyle," August 1, 2006. www. emaxhealth.com.

How Should Obesity Be Treated?

43. Louis Flancbaum, Erica Manfred, and Deborah Flancbaum, *The Doctor's Guide to Weight Loss Surgery*. New York: Bantam, 2003, p. 28.

44. Susan Okie, *Fed Up! Winning the War Against Childhood Obesity*. Washington, DC: Joseph Henry, 2005, p. 224.

45. Flancbaum, Manfred, and Flancbaum, *The Doctor's Guide to Weight Loss Surgery*, p. 29.

46. Abbott Laboratories, "How Meridia Works," 2007. www.meridia.net.

47. Roche Laboratories Inc., "Xenical at Work," 2007. www.xenical.com.

48. GlaxoSmithKline, Alli brochure, 2006.

49. Sanjay Gupta, "Buyer Beware," *Time*, June 4, 2007.

50. Liposuction.com, "Common and Minor Complications," 2007. www.liposuction.com.

51. Anne Underwood and Jerry Adler, "What You Don't Know About Fat," *Newsweek*, August 23, 2004.

52. Okie, *Fed Up!* p. 238.

53. Kaufman, *Diabesity*, p. 195.

54. Quoted in Flancbaum, Manfred, and Flancbaum, *The Doctor's Guide to Weight Loss Surgery*, p. 175.

List of Illustrations

List of Illustrations

Index

About the Author

Carrie Fredericks received her degree from Detroit's Wayne State University, majoring in English and minoring in general science studies. She has worked on many informational directories and edited several science and medical publications. She resides with her family in Michigan.